Diagnosis: Brain Tumor
My Acoustic Neuroma Story

C. Michael Miller

DEDICATION

This book is dedicated to the memory of Dr. Glenn G. Marinelli.
Thank you for everything.

CONTENTS

ACKNOWLEDGMENTS

This project wouldn't have ever existed without two groups of people: the people who helped me through my brain tumor experience and the people who helped me through the writing process. Of course, some were involved in both cases.

A very special thanks goes out to my amazing wife for always standing beside me, behind me, and in front of me, whether I deserved it or not. I appreciate the gentle encouragement through all of this. I'm a lucky guy.

Another special thanks goes out to three incredible doctors, my physical therapist, and all the wonderful people supporting them. To Dr. Marinelli, Dr. Kim, Dr. Jean, Danielle, and everyone involved with helping them do their incredible work- Thank you so much.

To Dad, Mom, Pat, and Bob- thank you for all the support.

Thanks to Bogey for all the great snuggles, and to GEGR, Throttle, Clutch, and all the foster kids for allowing me to give back in my own way.

Thank you to all my great friends for being so supportive and understanding.

And a huge thank you to Jim R. Miller, Pat Miller, Bob Segan, Pat Rouzer, Jim A. Miller, Charlotte, Mark, Joan Geer, and Ami- without whom this story would have ended up being the boring drivel it started out as.

INTRODUCTION

Since I wasn't allowed to move my head or upper body at all, I was watching my toes wiggle a little dance in my sneakers while I sang, in my head, the song that the Typewriter Guy used to sing on Sesame Street. *Nooooney, Noooney, Nooney, Noo... T. Toes.* I chuckled a little. I was in the middle of getting a cranial MRI scan and was watching my toes do their little dance in my sneakers in the angled mirror that I think was supposed to make me feel less claustrophobic. I just thought it was handy for keeping an eye on my toes while they wiggled and danced to the song I sang in my head. I'm guessing that's not what the company who designed the MRI machine really had in mind, but I wasn't worried about it.

A sudden movement in the smoked glass window beyond my feet caught my eye. The silhouette in the control room was pointing and gesturing at something. There were quickly other shadows that came over to gather around and see what had attracted the first silhouette's attention. My song faded off into nothing and my toes stopped dancing as the profile of a man wearing a tie came into view and started pointing and gesturing as well.

This can't be good, I thought. Pointing and gesturing during medical tests like an MRI is generally bad, even if it's just pointing done by silhouettes and shadows. Little did I know what the future held in store for me.

Part 1 - Diagnosis

1 – SUMMER 2008

You know that weird pressure that you get in your ears when you can't get the pressure to equalize on an airplane, or you have a head cold, or you go scuba diving? I had that pressure in just my left ear. It was driving me nuts. I have always been able to wiggle my jaw just right and do this thing with my tongue and get the pressure to equalize. I was doing the jaw thing a lot but I just couldn't get the feeling of pressure to go away. I also couldn't hear quite right out of that ear. All of the sounds I heard in that ear seemed really distant and thin. Everything sounded like faint AM radio.

I thought maybe it was wax build-up. Gross, right? But I had suffered from that sometimes as a kid. I remember our family doctor using a Waterpik machine to clean out my ears when that happened. I don't even think they still make those anymore. I'm not entirely convinced that it was the safest thing to stick in a kid's ears, either. But I will give it credit for being effective. The doctor would put warm water in it and something to loosen the gunk in my ears (vinegar maybe?). Then a nurse would hold a cup under my ear while the doctor went to town with the Waterpik. All manor of disgusting crud would get cleaned out of my ears and I would be able to hear again.

My wife, Kay, loves stories like this from my childhood. OK, she doesn't really love them, in fact I'm not sure she even really ever believes them. I don't care what she says, this particular story is completely true. And kind of disgusting at the same time.

I wasn't about to do anything like the Waterpik method on my own, so I went to the store and found the ear cleaning kits in the pharmacy aisle and purchased a couple different versions. It turns out they are mostly all the same: mineral oil goes in the ear to soak into compacted wax in order to loosen it, and then a squeeze ball to help rinse your ear out after you let the oil drain out. I used both of the kits, but neither of them helped at all. Nothing even came out. Now I was wondering if there was anything in there at all, or if everything was just packed in there really tight. Maybe it was time to go see a professional.

I think I'm a pretty typical person in that I really don't like going to doctors. It takes something pretty serious to get me to go. It's not really a fear thing, I don't think. OK, maybe it is a fear thing. Who knows? Kay and I didn't have a really spectacular Primary Care Provider at this point, anyway. We were both basically healthy people, so there just wasn't ever much need to find a great practice. Neither of us had ever seen an actual doctor at the Primary Care office we went to. We were always given appointments with one of the two nurse practitioners in the office. My wife and I were even lucky enough to have pretty high-end health insurance, so I really can't imagine how difficult it would have been to get an appointment with a doctor with little or no health insurance. I know the medical care situation in our nation is messed up, and I don't claim to know how to fix it, but I think you should be able to see a doctor when you go to the doctor's office. Our primary care provider at this point evidently seemed to feel differently. I sometimes wondered what all the doctors with their names painted on the door did all day if the nurse practitioners were the only ones seeing patients. My guess is that they have a really long running poker game going in some conference room. I finally couldn't stand the weird pressure in my ear and made an appointment with the nurse practitioner I usually saw.

I'm not sure why I kept going back to this particular nurse practitioner. Maybe I was just a glutton for punishment. She always had weird, kind of medieval remedies for things that seemed like they should have straight forward, scientific answers in modern medicine. The best example of that was the day that I hurt my ankle doing laundry. I was carrying a basket of dirty laundry down the steps from our second floor to the laundry room on the first floor. The basket blocked my view of the stairs and I missed the bottom step. Missing the step caused me to step awkwardly and very heavily on my right foot, which sent a shooting pain through my ankle. The pain was bad enough that I called our primary care provider and, to no particular surprise, ended up seeing the nurse practitioner. I figured she'd x-ray the ankle, brace it or put a cast on it, and then admonish me for being an idiot. No such luck. No x-ray, no brace, no cast. She told me to trace out each letter of the alphabet with my foot each day. What? Trace the alphabet? Why wouldn't we x-ray the stupid thing? I did get admonished for wearing shoes that she didn't feel were supportive enough. Years later that ankle now cracks and pops every morning when I walk down the stairs. Unfortunately, the lesson I learned wasn't to get a different Primary Care office; instead, I learned to be more careful doing laundry. I am such an idiot.

During this visit, the nurse practitioner examined my ear and found it to be completely clear all the way to the ear drum. The device with the light on it that doctors use to check out ears and noses got shoved in my ear. She couldn't find anything in my ear that could be causing my symptoms. Then the inspection device got shoved in my nose. I can honestly say that, given the choice, I preferred it shoved in my ear rather than my nose. That conical part that gets inserted isn't terribly comfortable on the nose, especially when it gets pulled up so the person holding it doesn't have to bother to ask me to tilt my head back. She did find that I had swollen sinuses that were most likely caused by allergies. That was her diagnosis for my problem: allergies. I was given a prescription for a nasal spray, and she told me to get an over-the-counter decongestant and anti-histamine. She also suggested I take more hot showers and make sure I was breathing in the steam through my nose. All of this along with doing the bit with the bowl of steaming hot water and a towel over your head to inhale the steam from that, too.

I wasn't overly impressed. First of all, I've had allergies all of my life. I remember being in Junior High School and waking up in the morning to a sneezing fit that would be at least fifteen or twenty sneezes long. I used to count them. Yes, I really was that cool. "Ah-Choo! One," and so on. The nasal spray the nurse practitioner prescribed was the same stuff that our family doctor prescribed for me back then. Really? Nasal sprays haven't gotten any better in twenty years? And what kind of archaic remedy is the whole "bowl of hot water and a towel" thing? I think I remember June Cleaver making the Beaver use that method. Come to think of it, I'm pretty sure she made Wally put a steak on his bruised face after a scuffle with Eddie Haskell, too. I wondered when the meat counter would join the bowl and towel as my prescribed medical treatments. But I figured I'd give it a try. You're supposed to be able to trust your medical professional, right? Turns out that I might have been giving a little more credit than was due in this case.

I took all the medications every day. I am not the best pill taker in the world, so this wasn't necessarily a lot of fun. There was usually a gagging incident or two during the week. I inhaled the steam in the shower. I will admit that I did not participate in the witchcraft with the bowl and towel. That was just too bizarre. The nasal spray hadn't improved in twenty years, it was some miserable crap. I didn't mind the anti-histamine or decongestant. I returned to see her a couple of months later when the medications ran out. I told her that, while I had never breathed so well in all my life, there was still the pressure in my ear. She yelled at me for not taking the stuff right. Or often enough. Or whatever. I quit paying attention when she started yelling at me. I had quit going to dentists for a stretch of almost ten years at one point because I hated getting yelled at for not flossing. I think everyone hates getting yelled at at the dentist. You do your best to keep your teeth basically healthy, then get berated by some dental technician for not flossing. It was so frustrating to go see this woman for help with my problem and have her yell at me! I needed professional medical help, and yet here's some old witchdoctor braying at me about how I wasn't using the twenty year old recipe of nasal spray correctly. I swear, if we had been in a spooky cave instead of the office and you put a tall, pointy hat on her, you'd wonder where her cauldron was. I was genuinely of the opinion that she could take her nasty nasal spray and her bowl of hot water and stick them in a closet in the witches' guild hall.

After she got done yelling at me, she suggested that my dogs were causing my allergies and I should get rid of them. The same dogs that we'd had starting with Rider in 2001 and never caused me any issues. I just stared at her. My wife and I don't have children. Well, not human children. Our two greyhounds were part of our family and I can assure you that they weren't going anywhere. Basically, I left with no more information than when I came in months earlier. I did have the added benefit of being frustrated and angry at my medical "professional."

I'm being too hard on her, you say? Do you really think so? I think one of the most professional things that any expert in a field, medicine being a perfect example, can do is say the words, "I don't know." Instead, I'm stuck with some hack that is yelling at me and telling me I should take my dogs to the shelter. Or put them in her potion. Had she just consulted with a real doctor at this point, we might have been saved a lot of trouble moving forward. She didn't. I'd pay for it in the future. Yes, I could have done things differently.

I could have insisted that I see one of the real doctors in the practice. Or I could have immediately made an appointment with a different doctor somewhere else to get a second opinion. I didn't. And again, I'd pay for it in the future.

2 - SUMMER 2009

A year went by. I hadn't done anything else to try to nail down the source of my symptoms. I just tried to ignore it and hope it got better. That didn't work any better than the witchcraft. The pressure and hearing loss were getting worse. I was doing the trick with my jaw constantly, but it wasn't working anymore. My jaw muscles were constantly sore from all the manipulation, and the weird pressure was driving me up the wall. Fast.

I decided the time had come to try again to get it fixed. I called to make an appointment with an Ear, Nose, and Throat specialist who had an office in my local area. They didn't have any openings soon in the local office, so I agreed to an appointment about ninety minutes away in their Bethesda office. I was going to see a nurse practitioner again. I was a little put off after my last nurse practitioner experience, but I was desperate at this point. The nurse practitioner I saw in the new practice was much better. She seemed actually concerned about me and didn't look like she was about to start yelling. We went through a battery of hearing tests and a full examination. She found that my hearing was significantly compromised (my wife could have told her that), and that the ear was still clear and my sinuses were still swollen. She put me on another set of medications based around decongestants and anti-histamines, but with a much better nasal spray this time. She definitely thought that I should see one of the Ear, Nose, and Throat doctors in the practice, so she made me an appointment with a doctor in their office near my house. This had been a much better experience. Telling me that she wasn't sure what was wrong and that I should see a doctor from their office was very reassuring. No sign of any flying broomsticks here. I chastised myself for all the time I wasted with the previous practice.

I was pleasantly surprised with the doctor's office when I arrived at the appointment in their branch near my house. Instead of a big, fluorescent bulb lit waiting area full of sniffling kids, the waiting area here was warmly lit, had a coffee pot on a counter in the corner, and was downright peaceful.

My ENT specialist appointment was with Dr. Glenn Marinelli. Dr. Marinelli was an easy going, middle-aged guy who was very personable. I felt genuinely comfortable explaining my symptoms to him while he listened attentively. This was such a relief after my experience in 2008. I was seeing a real doctor who listened to me and was really concerned about my problem. We went through another full examination and battery of testing. Stick the inspection tool in my ear, put on these headphones and raise your hand when you hear a sound, and the rest of the drill. Everything in my ear was still unobstructed, but my hearing was getting worse while the pressure was getting more aggravating. Dr. Marinelli was plainly concerned over the fact that the symptoms in my left ear were so bad while my right ear was just fine. I could tell he really wanted to help me and was just wracking his brain for an answer. He said he was going to do more research and try to figure it out for our next appointment. In the meantime, he wanted me to get an MRI of my head done in order to eliminate a really rare tumor that was possible, but not likely to be the culprit. I felt really encouraged when I left my appointment with Dr. Marinelli. It seemed to me that I had found the right person to help me.

As interesting as this part of the story might be (or might not be, as it were), have you noticed that I haven't mentioned anything about what was going on in the rest of my life during this time period? It wasn't all just medical appointments, whether it felt that way or not, but all we have really talked about so far is the process of trying to get these weird symptoms diagnosed. I went ahead and scheduled the MRI for the following Monday as kind of an afterthought.

It turns out that I was right in the middle of the worst week of my life. I understand that this is a phrase often used just for dramatic effect, but in this case it is absolutely true. I had seen Dr. Marinelli early in the week on Monday or Tuesday and had my MRI scheduled for Monday of the next week.

One of our retired racing greyhounds, Rider, had been given a bone cancer diagnosis earlier that year and was slowly dying. His quality of life had taken a recent turn for the worse and so we had decided to let him go on that Thursday. That was a really emotional day. Rider had only run one race in his career- he came in last- after which he was put up for adoption. I guess that's what happens to a dog whose race notes for that single race were simply: OOP. Out Of Picture. Poor Rider was kind of a scaredy-cat, and we're guessing that he came out of the starting box and was terrified by all the noise and commotion that surrounds a dog race. So he had been with us since just before he turned two years old in 2002. Now, seven fun and love-filled years later, we had to say goodbye.

That trip to the vet made Thursday terrible. It was just so sad to say goodbye. How could it be that we had to make this decision for the goofy dog that didn't know what to do with the squirrel he had caught in the yard one time? The poor guy had just stood there all proud of himself with the terrified squirrel in his jaws, that proceeded to bite him on the nose. He figured out that shaking the squirrel was a good idea after it bit him, but it was so interesting to watch an eighty-five pound hunting machine not know what to do when he caught his prey. They never taught him that lesson at greyhound racing school. With memories like that, it was inevitable that Kay and I were emotional wrecks. The kisses that he reached up and gave me while I held him didn't help my emotional state, either.

On Friday our computer died. It had been acting up for a while and chose that particular day to just not bother to boot up at all. So what? We were completely cut off from the world. No internet, no email, no nothing. We hadn't made the move to smart phones yet, so we were back to the days of phone calls to contact people. I was fit to be tied when I couldn't do any reading on the internet about the possible tumor that the doctor thought I might have. All weekend I would think of a question about something and be just about to head upstairs to the home office to check on it when I'd remember that I couldn't. So I'd just stand at the stairs and be frustrated. I think the banister learned a couple of new phrases consisting of all four letter

9

words that weekend. The only thing to do was order a new laptop over the weekend. So Kay took care of that with HP over the phone. Our new machine would arrive in about a week. All of which leads us into Monday.

I had never had an MRI before, but I figured it couldn't be too bad. After all, I had seen them on the medical drama shows on TV and it never looked bad there. The very enigmatic doctor would be trying to solve the mystery of the elusive diagnosis and gain some amazing insight while asking the patient some inane question during their MRI. It actually sounds kind of fun when you put it that way. Everybody loves those shows! Armed with that stellar bit of information I didn't think there was anything to be nervous about, so I just wasn't nervous.

I drove to the local radiology facility located in the building across the parking lot from the movie theater and supermarket for my appointment. The local gym had also moved into the same building so, on my way in the front door, I passed all the super muscle jock types coming out from their work-outs. It left me feeling a bit emasculated to have all those guys with their big muscles walking around while I was walking into the building a good forty pounds overweight and completely out of shape.

I felt even more out of place as soon as I opened the door to the radiology office. The waiting room was filled with pregnant women and little kids. Why was the waiting area filled with pregnant women? I couldn't figure it out. Then it occurred to me that ultrasound was a radiology process. Oh. Right. OK. I checked in at the front desk and they asked me to fill out a questionnaire. No problem. I went to find a spot to sit. The waiting area was not quite half full, but because of the personal space requirements of the American general public, the only seats open were all between pregnant women. I know that pregnant women have a mystique about them- that they are somehow these glowing, wonderful, maternal sirens that sooth troubled souls. I'm sure that's true in some settings or in some other world that I don't spend much time in. But when you're the only man under the age of seventy-five in a room full of pregnant women, they seem more like angry bears protecting their den. Maybe it was just my imagination. It seemed odd though, since a similar waiting room full of men at the car parts shop would like nothing more than to have a reasonably attractive woman come sit near them. Heck, I wasn't a bad looking guy. OK, I had a few extra pounds in a nice paunch, but it seemed like that would make me seem harmless. I had a nice tan from all the time I spent outside, and I always had a cool haircut. Evidently there was a significant difference between how dudes at the parts store felt about attractive women and how pregnant women at the radiology lab felt about reasonable looking guys. I finally managed to find a seat between a couple of ladies that seemed less likely to maul me to death than some of the others, and started filling out the requested paperwork.

The questionnaire was very specific and detailed. There were several pages of check-lists to go over and a whole host of in-depth questions with plenty of space to go into detail in your answers. I wasn't running for President, why does the MRI place need to know what my hobbies are? Let's see, I enjoy sailing, riding my bicycle, playing my guitar on the boat, and trying new ethnic food recipes. No, I didn't have Tuberculosis, thank you very much. Yes, my welding skills are proficient- but I work as the manager for our vacation rental house, so I wasn't applying for a job in steel fabrication. What was the story with these questions? I wondered how many of the pregnant momma bears held an up-to-date welding certification. It turned out that all of these questions, with the exception of my curiosity about the number of pregnant women holding welding certs, would be answered in good time.

After I finished with the questionnaire, I sat back down to watch incredibly bad daytime TV talk shows that everybody else seemed mesmerized by. This was that point where throwing a chair at some poor man who refused to get a paternity test was still mildly popular with audiences. A nurse wearing dark maroon scrubs came out of the back and called my name, saving me from the inevitable audience Q&A session on the television. I followed her back where they showed me into a dressing area and handed me a packaged gown. A gown? Really? First a bunch of "Chet" guys in the parking lot, then a room full of angry looking pregnant women, and now a hospital gown? This wasn't anything like the cool medical dramas on TV! At no point did I feel like L.L. Cool J's character from his guest appearance on *House* while I was changing into my gown. I came out of the changing room and the nurse showed me to a locker area where she asked me to put my clothes, my wristwatch, and my wedding band. I put in my rolled-up jeans and shirt, placed my wedding ring and watch on top, closed the door, and clicked the padlock closed. I followed the nurse into a fairly large, dimly lit room. All of the lighting was focused in the center of the room where she politely asked me to stand. Standing there in the lit area of an otherwise darkened room made me think of several one-person stage shows I had seen. Broadway style one-person shows, not those other ones; I wasn't covered in glitter, nor was there a pole.

I had filled out the questionnaire pretty honestly when I had checked in. That presented a bit of a problem because of my answers to the questions in the section asking if I had ever done any work with metal or welding. I'm not a welder or machinist or anything, but I've done a fair amount of welding while working on various hobby projects and had just finished up a boat project in the spring that involved a lot of metal grinding. The radiologist was concerned that I might have tiny metal fragments embedded in my skin or eyes that could present a real danger during the MRI process. Magnetic Resonance... Oh yeah, right! Now all those questions about my hobbies and metalworking history made sense. My lack of understanding might seem naive, and I suppose it probably was, but keep in mind that my previous health-care professional was the lady stirring the cauldron while I spelled out the alphabet with my broken ankle. Plus, all the pregnant ladies had been making me nervous, so I wasn't even thinking very clearly when I had filled out the paperwork. I had been too busy trying to stave off the urge to go find bacon and pickle-flavored ice cream for the people sitting around me to pay much attention.

I spent the next hour or so getting cranial X-rays done. There in the dark room, they led me to a head immobilizer with a chin rest and asked me to place my head in it. Then the nurse left the room and a set of cross-hairs appeared on my head. It reminded me a lot of the opening scene from the old 1970's *Incredible Hulk* TV show where Bill Bixby had the circle and hash marks light up his face before he's overcome by gamma rays. Yes, I know I watch too much TV. I was getting more and more nervous as it became clear that getting my MRI wasn't going to be anything like what I had imagined. But envisioning myself in some of these television shows kept my brain occupied and helped me to keep most of the nervous tension at bay.

I appreciated the care that the radiology lab professionals took to be sure I wouldn't be injured by the MRI machine sending a metal fragment rocketing out of my eye or something, but it did build a little bit of anxiety about the whole process in me forcing me to get into even more detail about Bixby's gamma ray overdose in my mind. I imagined myself in that fancy motorized chair he had, turning this way and that to get the cross-hairs focused, while the piano music built tension and the guy with the cool voice talked about the dangers of having the MRI machine pull a tiny bit of metal through my brain. My x-ray session was over before I had the chance to imagine myself splitting my mauve bell-bottom pants or somebody decided that the dark green color I was painted was too frightening for young children. Someday my vivid imagination was going to get me in trouble.

Once they decided I wasn't a walking load of shrapnel, the nurse in the maroon scrubs took me into the MRI area. The machine itself was really big. It was about the size of a panel truck. The room that held it was huge! It was not quite as big as the gymnasium in the small town elementary school that I attended as a child in Minnesota, but it was very close. In fact, I would bet that the overall square footage of the MRI room was bigger. It was chilly in the room, but the walls were painted a nice, warming, light yellow color and even the glass panels in the ceiling were painted to look like a sky with puffy clouds in it. I guess that was supposed to be relaxing. It didn't really work for me. I wasn't a nervous mess or anything, but I definitely was kind of uncomfortable. There was also a large, "one way mirror" type of smoked glass window in the wall facing the front of the machine. I guessed it was the control room.

The nurses had me lie down on the machine's table and put a pillow under my knees so that I'd be comfortable, obviously a technique learned from dealing with all the pregnant women, and I was given a pair of purple foam earplugs. Earplugs were at least something I understood well. Years of playing in various rock & roll bands and working out on the airport tarmac for a major express shipping company had left me well versed in their use. Had I known I was going to need them, I would have brought my custom fit musician plugs since they are far more comfortable than the disposable foam plugs I was given. I rolled the earplugs to compress them and inserted them in each ear, holding my finger tip against each one while it expanded. The nurse even offered me a blanket, but I politely declined. I had my nerves to keep me warm. I was just lying there comfortably and starting to relax. Maybe this wouldn't be so bad, after all. Perhaps all the nerves and classic TV show immersion had been overkill. The nurse gave me a button with a plastic tube that led down to my right. She explained it was my panic button. I should use it at any point if I needed help or got too uncomfortable. The presence of the panic button warned me to keep the TV references close at hand. Next, she slid what I can only describe as a cylindrical cage down over my head. It had a mirror mounted in it right over my eyes at an angle that let me see down towards my feet. I guessed it was for people who were uncomfortable in tight spaces. That seemed to me like a really thoughtful solution to what was sure to be a common problem. I wasn't convinced that it was really necessary for me, though. The table then slid into the vertical, donut shaped tube of the MRI machine and the nurses and technicians left the room.

I am not too proud to admit that the mirror was a good idea. I had never had any issues with claustrophobia before and don't really mind close spaces at all, but I was still a little uncomfortable. I can't imagine how terrified someone with a real bad case of claustrophobia would be, even with the mirror. I would guess there was some Valium or something nearby for those people, just in case. Given that I was getting an MRI of my head done, my line of sight was inside the ring of the machine the entire time. I had also wondered about why they had given me the ear plugs. A woman's calm voice came over an intercom to make sure that I was ready to start and had my panic button in hand. Sure, let's start! The machine was unbelievably loud, which explained the earplugs. It made all sorts of mechanical noises. It sounded like I was in a large factory in the early 1900's with all the buzzing, clicking, and whirring. It wasn't quite as loud as somebody's screaming guitar solo or a 727 jet airplane taxiing in, but it was close. I did my best to settle in and relax, since this would take a while. Well, as relaxed as I could get without moving at all.

They had told me that the first part of the process would take about thirty minutes. About twenty minutes into the scan, I noticed a commotion from the silhouettes in the tech room via my mirror. The movement had distracted me from the infantile fascination I was having with using the angled mirror to watch my toes dance in my sneakers to the song that the Typewriter Guy used to sing on Sesame Street back in the 1970's. Since I couldn't move my head or shoulders, I had been compensating and keeping myself busy by singing that little song in my head while I alternated lifting my big toes to poke at the mesh top on my shoes. All done in rhythm to the silly, happy tune that was warbling around in my head- *Nooooney, noooney, nooney, noo... T. Toes.* The silhouettes in the control room were pointing and gesturing and gathering around what I assumed to be a monitor. My fun little song sort of trailed off while I watched through the smoked glass, though I would guess my toes kept their rhythm going for a while but I wasn't paying attention anymore.

A silhouette with a tie appeared and looked to be examining the monitor. It's amazing how much of a vague understanding of things you can glean from just silhouettes. I gathered something was not quite right, given all the pointing and the fact that they found somebody in a tie to come in and look. The first round of imaging finished up and the machine shut down. The nurse came in and moved me out of the machine in order to inject some contrast dye into my arm for the next round. She didn't say a word about the excitement in the control room and I was too distracted by the needle to ask. I don't really like needles very well, but I just averted my eyes and the nurse did a great job of getting the injection done quickly and painlessly.

How could I have been distracted from a bunch of people pointing at something while I was getting an MRI? Easy, just let me explain just how much I don't like needles. I had a small surgical procedure done in the fall of 2001 to remove a couple of cysts from my scalp. When I was having my IV inserted, I was smart enough to look the other way. The nurse seemed done with the insertion, so I brought my gaze back up from the far wall. It turned out that the nurse wasn't quite finished yet, since he hadn't covered the insertion site at all. I turned sheet white and started to faint right there on the gurney. My wife was there and she recognized the issue and told the nurse who promptly pumped me full of happy juice and tilted my gurney so that my legs were up in the air and my head was down low. Ever since, I try to warn anybody with a needle about my fear. At least we don't ever have to worry about me being a heroin junkie, right?

After the dye injection, I went back into the machine for about another fifteen minutes of scans. I felt like someone's favorite holiday baked goods recipe: prop with pillow, insert earplugs, bake for thirty minutes- then remove from oven, inject with contrast dye and put back for an additional fifteen minutes. There weren't any happy tunes or silly toes this time since the second round of scanning with the contrast dye led to even more pointing and gesturing in the control room. Hmmm, I thought, all that pointing and gesturing and calling in men in ties can't have been good. I tried to think of a time when pointing and gesturing hadn't been bad. I couldn't come up with anything. First, I tried sailing scenarios: pirates, giant waves, and you could go all the way back to Odysseus navigating the Scylla and Charybdis. No good pointing there. Tornadoes? No. That train bearing down on us? Nope. There just weren't any examples that I could think of where pointing like that wasn't a bad thing.

When the scan was finished, they took me out of the machine and back to the dressing area and I got changed. I was glad to get back into street clothes. It made things seem less scary. One of the nurses had the films ready for me when I finished up getting dressed and I was told to take them to my doctor's office. Luckily, Dr. Marinelli's office was just down the street so I dropped them off on the way home. I didn't really give it all that much thought other than to describe the MRI process to my wife. I didn't mention to her the part about all the pointing and gesturing from the control room. I guess that was a bit of an oversight on my part. It wasn't an oversight that scored me any brownie points with her later on.

We were still reeling from Thursday's trip to the vet to say goodbye to our Rider, so Monday evening we took our other greyhound, Bogey, for a walk. A warm June evening made for a wonderful time to all go for a walk together. We had been spending so much time over the past couple of weeks paying attention to Rider that poor Bogey hadn't gotten as much attention as he should have. Making time to do the little extra things with him was important for him to be sure we still loved him, and was important for us to help cope with the loss of Rider. It was also a good chance for me to tell Kay all about my entertaining day with the fearsome pregnant women, the Bill Bixby x-ray session, and my time in the MRI tube. I'll be honest- the oversight of not telling her about the pointing and gesturing silhouettes was just that. There was so much going on my head that evening that I just plain old forgot about it. It could have also been my brain coping with what I had seen the people doing in that control room by just sectioning it away somewhere deep.

I got a call from Dr. Marinelli's office first thing on Tuesday morning. Could I come in today and see him? Sure thing. I asked what he had available in his schedule. They told me I didn't need an appointment, he'd make time for me whenever I came in. So I had a bite to eat for breakfast, drove up to the office and told the receptionist that I was there to see the doctor. I didn't even get a chance to sit down to wait. Dr. Marinelli came down the hall and politely ushered me into his office. Much like the pointing and gesturing during the MRI, I couldn't think of any point where a doctor would just drop everything to come out and kindly walk you back to his office that ended in anything good. I was right on this account, too.

Dr. Marinelli put the MRI films up on a light board mounted on the wall. He then described the basics of what we were seeing in the images. There were several different images from two angles. The first angle showed images as if you were looking down on the top of my head. The MRI process allows them to make images as if it were a slice of whatever they were looking at. So I could see each level starting with the top of my head down through the levels of my eyes, nose, mouth, etc. The same was true of the other angle except front to back. He pointed out landmarks like the skull, eyes, brain stem, brain (I couldn't resist the inevitable joke about proving to my wife that I actually had a brain), nasal cavity, etc... "Mr. Miller, do you see the large white mass right there?" Ummm, yeah? "That's why I had you get an MRI. It's a tumor called an Acoustic Neuroma. It's a benign tumor, but it is pushing on your auditory nerve and is causing your discomfort and hearing loss. It is quite large as these go, and as you can see here, it is also pushing up against your cerebellum and brain stem. You are going to need to have surgery to have it removed." I'm sure that during any patient's diagnosis of any major medical issue they have had a similar conversation with their doctor. I'm also guessing the reaction is pretty standard.

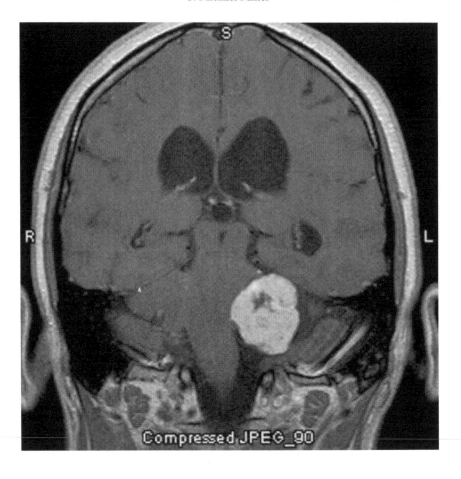

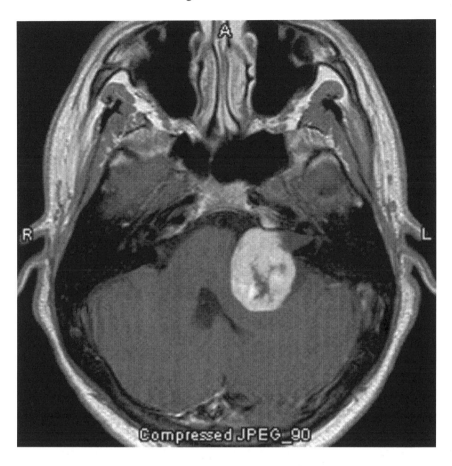

I was floored. What did he just say? Oh, crap- surgery? He went on to explain what type of surgery was typical and that his guess was that there would be a three or four week recovery from the surgery. I was barely listening. I remember looking at him while he was talking to me and all I could think was, *Did he just say I have a brain tumor? I think he did.* Dr. Marinelli said that he knew a surgeon up at Georgetown University Hospital that specialized in these things (what did he call it again? I couldn't remember. An Acoustic what?). He would be glad to call and try to get me set up with an appointment with the surgeon at Georgetown so I wouldn't have to wait. After we had gotten done with the conversation about going up to see the surgeon at Georgetown, our meeting was pretty much over. But before I left, Dr. Marinelli looked me in the eye and said, "Mr. Miller, go to a specialty hospital for this- don't let a local doctor drill a hole in your head." I just nodded, but it was pretty damned sage advice.

I would like to take just a minute to say a special thank you to Dr. Glenn Marinelli. Without his expertise and experience, I probably would have kept chasing this diagnosis around for months or years to come. He had used his skill and experience to help us look in the right direction for an answer. If the nurse practitioner had done this over a year earlier, things would have been so much simpler. I was just glad that I had found Dr. Marinelli when I did. As we'll see later, his diagnosis probably saved my life. Thanks Doc, I owe you one. Big time.

I called my wife to tell her about all this on the way home. I don't remember too much else of that day. It's all just a blur. I do remember sitting at the kitchen table with the envelope containing my MRI images sitting in front of me. I would carefully take out each film in turn and hold it up to the light to see the image of the tumor in my head. In one scan, the tumor would seem very small where the film showed the very top of it, then each subsequent scan would show the cross-sections getting larger and larger until we saw it in all its 3.9cm of glory. I couldn't believe it. That giant white blob was in my head. I showed the MRI films to Kay when she got home from work that night. We held them up to the light in the kitchen and I pointed at the big white thing in my noggin and I said, "well *here's* my problem" or something like that. Neither one of us really understood what was happening yet, so we figured we'd just do what needed to be done. What else is there to do? Oh, and I did tell her the joke about proof of me actually having a brain. Seriously, who can resist a temptation like that? Definitely not the guy who was humming a little song for his toes to dance to while he was getting an MRI the day before. I'm not sure she thought my joke was funny.

We've just relived the worst week of my life. A doctor's appointment where we're still trying to figure out what is causing my issues on Monday or Tuesday. Letting our dying dog go on Thursday. Having our computer crash on Friday. Getting an MRI on Monday and finding out that I had a big brain tumor on Tuesday, just to round the week out. Such fun. How do you top a stellar week like that?

3 – WHAT NOW?

With the help of Dr. Marinelli's office, I had an appointment at Georgetown University Hospital to see the surgeon he had recommended. I had lived in and around the Washington, DC metro area since 1996, but I was always fascinated with spending time in Georgetown. On the way to the hospital, we drove over the Key Bridge into town- dumping us right out on "M" Street with all of its restaurants and high end clothing stores. Few people, even residents of Washington, realize that the point where the bridge takes you into Georgetown is just yards from the location of the home of the bridge's namesake, Francis Scott Key. He was living there in the year 1814 when he traveled to Baltimore to negotiate the release of American prisoners during the War of 1812. The British held Key on board the ship where the negotiations took place throughout the night of the bombardment of Fort McHenry to prevent him from passing along valuable information about troop and ship placements to the Americans. He was moved by the sight of the American flag flying defiantly over Fort McHenry the next morning. On his way back into Baltimore he wrote the poem that would later become the American National Anthem. Unfortunately, after being dismantled in preparation to move the house, all the pieces of the structure were lost. Its location remains a mystery to this day.

We turned left off of "M" onto 34th Street and drove up through some of the more residential sections of Georgetown. We passed by very pricey town houses and incredibly expensive single-family homes. Few of them had off-street parking, leaving the curbs of the narrow streets jammed with parked, high-end SUV's. We made the turn onto the Georgetown University Medical campus and parked in the underground garage.

My wife and I weren't really sure what to expect as we went to the appointment in the department of Otolaryngology (Ear, Nose, and Throat) with Dr. Kim. I was really glad that Kay went along with me to this appointment, and I'd suggest you have a loved one go with you as well if you are ever facing something like this. Having someone at these early appointments with you will help to make sure that you absorb all the information that will be presented to you. We walked through the medical building; it looked a little older than some of the other buildings but was still very well maintained. We found Dr. Kim's office and went inside.

Having my wife with me made me far less nervous in the waiting area than I had been at the MRI appointment. It also helped that the waiting area wasn't full of hostile looking pregnant women. The waiting area had a small nook off to one side that was wallpapered with children's designs and there were plenty of toys and books to keep kids busy. I thought that was a super idea in an office that surely saw a large number of sick kids. Since Kay was with me, I refrained from going in and playing with the toys. I got checked in and gave the receptionist the MRI films. Dr. Kim's staff was great. Everyone from the person who checked me in at the front desk, all the way through the person at billing and everyone in between, were very friendly and helpful.

I was called back by a nurse who suggested that Kay could come back and join us as well. The nurse took me to a scale in the hallway and got my height and weight measurements, then we went to an exam room. I sat in the exam chair, which was remarkably similar to a chair in a dentist office, while Kay sat on a stool off to the side. The nurse went through a few questions, and she took my pulse and my blood pressure. I asked how my blood pressure was, and she replied that it was just fine. I thought that was surprising considering why I was there to see the doctor. Then she left and said that Dr. Kim would be in shortly to review my situation with us.

Dr. Hung Jeffrey Kim was a slightly built man with a pleasant smile and a very friendly demeanor. He seemed to be about ten years older than Kay and I. He introduced himself and explained

that he had examined the MRI images and he agreed with Dr.
Marinelli's assessment that surgery would be the best course of
action in dealing with the tumor. He explained that because the
tumor was so large (3.9cm), it needed to be removed surgically as
soon as possible. Acoustic Neuroma tumors can range in size from
the tiny, measured in millimeters, to the large, which are measured in
centimeters. They are rarely much over 4cm, so my tumor fell into
the upper end of the size range. Remember when I said that Dr.
Marinelli probably saved my life? As he examined me and looked
more at the MRI images, Dr. Kim was shocked that the tumor hadn't
already affected my facial nerve and he even seemed surprised that I
still had full use of my faculties. Holy. Crap. His surprise stemmed
from the size and location of the tumor. It was so big, and pushing
on such critical stuff in my head that he was amazed that it hadn't
screwed something up other than my hearing and pressure sensation
in my ear. So all that time that I had wasted on allergy medications
and witchcraft had been letting my tumor grow larger to the point
that a specialist like Dr. Kim was surprised that I could still feel my
face. Wonderful.

I wasn't expecting the doctor to be surprised that I could still feel
my face on one side. Nor was I expecting anyone to be worried
about the tumor affecting my quality of life. I didn't have a full
understanding yet of the physiology involved with my tumor, so for
him to be surprised that I still had feeling and movement on the left
side of my face left me feeling a little nervous. How are you
supposed to react to a statement like that? I just nodded and assured
him that I could feel his fingers touching my cheek and made all the
funny facial expressions he asked me to. I was still just kind of
along for the ride at the time. I felt like everything up to this point
was really happening around me rather than happening to me. Even
though I had been surprised and nervous about the diagnosis, none of
the reality of the situation had caught up to me yet. Don't worry,
though, it will catch up to me quickly and without mercy in just a
minute. No amount of the "Nooooney, noooney, nooney, noo" song
or dancing toes was going to get me out of this one.

Dr. Kim explained that he worked as part of a team with a neuro-
surgeon at Georgetown on surgeries to remove these tumors. He
said that they did about three or four Acoustic Neuroma surgeries
each month. Kay and I thought that was great news. We felt like we

had come to the right place and were talking to the right people to get this taken care of. Acoustic Neuroma wasn't treated as a rare or surprising condition here at Georgetown. The realization that Dr. Marinelli had sent me someplace where people could help me took so much of the pressure off emotionally, it was amazing. Once I had found a doctor who knew what to look for in Dr. Marinelli, he had helped me find a path where I could trust all the people involved.

Dr. Kim decided to see if I could get on the other surgeon's schedule for that same day and so he pulled out his two-way text pager and sent the other doctor a message. He worked really hard to get me an appointment right then to go see the neuro-surgeon, Dr. Walter Jean. Again, I think that this really shows that I had come to the right place. The effort Dr. Kim put into getting me shoehorned in Dr. Jean's schedule that same day really showcased the dedication and concern that the Georgetown doctors (and I'm sure the same is true for doctors all over) have for their patients, even a new patient like me. But, unfortunately, Dr. Jean's schedule was just too full that day. We would have to come see him another time. I sat there watching all of this with a sense of disbelief. Dr. Kim seemed really disappointed that he couldn't get me in to see Dr. Jean. I still just didn't understand the hurry. I could just make an appointment and come see him another time, right? Especially since this whole thing is just happening around me while I watch.

Dr. Kim pulled up a stool and sat down. He began describing the surgical process that would best suit the removal of my tumor to my wife and me. I was going to have a trans-labyrinth (trans-lab) approach surgery. He wanted us to understand what was going to happen and what the surgical protocol would be. I thought this was a great idea, since it seemed to me that being armed with that information would help us make good decisions as this process went along. Information is always the best tool to have in your arsenal, right? I was wrong. It wasn't a good idea at all. Dr. Kim reached up to his head and traced a curve on his scalp above his ear and got as far as, "We'll start by cutting off your ear..." when I passed out. Right there in the examination chair. I got really hot all of the sudden, the room spun erratically, and I started to get tunnel vision. I think I made some attempt to get out of the chair, though that might have been my imagination. Then, whoosh, I was out.

That was the exact moment that this whole situation began to happen to me rather than around me. As I described earlier, everything up to that point seemed distant and removed like someone was telling me about it. Maybe it would be better described as having someone telling me about it all happening to somebody else that I had a lot in common with. It had all been happening to the imaginary me. Now it was happening to the real me. The me that sang stupid songs and watched way too much television. The me that had ignored the symptoms in hopes that they'd go away on their own so I wouldn't have to go back and get yelled at by that witch-doctor of a nurse practitioner. The me that was unconscious in an examination chair.

When I came to, I found myself reclined in the exam chair and my wife holding a damp paper towel on my forehead. The smell of the damp brown paper towel reminded me of good old Madison Elementary School again. I remembered when we used to fold that same type of paper towel up into squares, soak it with water, and throw it up to stick on the twelve foot ceilings in the boys lavatory. It's weird the stuff you remember when you wake up after a shock like I had. I looked up to see Kay's upside down face telling me it would be OK. A nurse was rubbing my arms to improve circulation and I could hear Dr. Kim asking someone to find him an ice pack for me. I was mortified. Had I really just passed out in the doctor's office? I was never going to live this one down. Wait- did he say he was going to cut off my ear? Whoa. Fainting was embarrassing, but I think that's a natural reaction to someone telling you that they're going to cut off your ear. They weren't going to cut it all the way off, just the top part and fold it down, but we'll get to all those details later. For now, Dr. Kim, Kay, and I decided that maybe we could just go through a generalized description of the surgical process. Perhaps we didn't really need all that information after all, right at that particular moment in time.

They got me a drink of water and got my blood pressure back up to a point where I could sit up comfortably again. Dr. Kim gave me a few minutes to compose myself before we continued. He proceeded to explain to us that I would come in for surgery early one morning, they would take the tumor out, I would probably have some temporary facial paralysis after, then I would recover in the hospital for about a week. I didn't pass out this time, but Dr. Kim looked really nervous as he was telling me all this stuff. I don't blame him at all. I know doctors and nurses see all sorts of strange things, but I'm not sure Dr. Kim was used to having patients pass out in his office.

When he asked, kind of nervously, if I had any questions, I asked if we could just put this off until winter. There was a lot of sailing to be done yet that summer. There were big regattas in July and September, and we were planning to do a lot of cruising on our boat during August and through the fall. Surely this whole surgery thing could wait until the off-season, right? Isn't that how pro athletes scheduled their surgical stuff? I certainly wasn't a pro athlete, but why not use them as an excuse to put this fiasco off for a little while. If I was going to have surgery, I wasn't going to let it affect all the fun stuff that I had planned for the rest of the summer. Dr. Kim was adamant about getting everything ready to have the surgery take place as soon as possible. I was assured that it could not wait because of the size and location of the tumor. He suggested that we call Dr. Jean's office as soon as we could to get an appointment to continue the process.

On a scale of one to ten, I would call my overall feelings about the outcome of that appointment: crappy. The appointment itself had been fine, if you excuse my very masculine fainting spell. Kay and I both really liked Dr. Kim and felt like he was definitely the person we should be talking to. I was not so thrilled about the realities of this getting in the way of the things I did for fun. But Kay did her best to convince me of how important this was on our way to the garage to get the car.

We called Dr. Jean's office while we were on the way home to get an appointment set up to see him. His staff found us a spot in his calendar for a few days later. Dr. Jean is a neuro-surgeon at Georgetown and the Acoustic Neuroma surgery is one of his specialties, teamed with Dr. Kim.

When we went back up to Georgetown for the appointment in the neuro-surgery department, we could tell that we were dealing with another top notch organization. The walls of the waiting area were filled with framed articles about the department from different magazines, newspapers, and medical journals along with several photos and thank-you letters from high visibility patients. There was not a children's area in the waiting room, so I wasn't even allowed to be tempted. I sat and read through old issues of People magazine.

Blech. It wasn't quite as ridiculous as the daytime TV I had watched before my MRI appointment, but it was close.

Dr. Jean had a very disarming personality that made him seem just like a regular guy, even though he actually was a brain surgeon. He had a great, dry sense of humor, which really put us at ease during the appointment. He invited us into one of the nicest exam rooms I had ever seen, and we sat down and he talked about his role in the tumor removal surgery and again stressed the need for this thing to come out as soon as possible due to its size.

I had done some research into different treatment options since our appointment with Dr. Kim a few days earlier and asked some questions about focused radiation treatments. I had read about a couple of different methods that used a very concentrated radiation to do pinpoint removal of tumors like mine without the need for invasive surgery and with few of the side effects of more traditional radiation treatments. Dr. Jean explained that my particular tumor was just too large to for any of those methods to be effective. Patients in my age range also sometimes developed issues stemming from the radiation later in life, so they preferred to use those on people who were a little older. We also discussed some of the generalities of what we could expect during the recovery process. Those included the loss of hearing in my left ear, which wasn't a huge deal since I had lost a lot of it over the past couple of years of symptoms anyway, some temporary facial paralysis on the left side of my face, and we'd go from there.

When Dr. Jean was finished he said, "This is the point where most people ask for a second opinion." Who would want a second opinion? These two doctors obviously knew their business very well. We couldn't think of anything we might gain by seeking another opinion, and so we told him that there was just no need for a second opinion. I guess we could have gone to another hospital and talked to other surgeons, but I think they probably would have told us the same basic things. He suggested we go ahead and get the surgery scheduled. He would reserve a surgery theater for as soon as possible. Again, he seemed concerned that we get things scheduled right away just like Dr. Kim had. There were two reasons for their desire to have the surgery on the schedule as soon as possible. First, Dr. Jean seemed to agree with Dr. Kim's assessment that I was right on the verge of the tumor having a very negative impact on me. The other reason was that Dr. Jean was going to be attending a conference out of town in a few weeks. He wanted to be sure that he would be around for the first part of my recovery after the surgery.

What minor details might we have glossed over to be sure I didn't pass out again, you ask? Good question. And don't worry, I won't pass out. The Trans-lab approach goes through the inner ear. Do you remember the Semicircular Canals with all the loops in your inner ear from your Junior High School biology or health class? That's part of the labyrinth they are talking about. I would lose my hearing in my left ear because of the damage done to the labyrinth area during the surgical procedure. Dr. Kim would start the surgery by cutting my scalp around the top half of my ear, folding it down like a flap. They would then drill a hole in my skull to accommodate the rest of the surgery. Next, Dr. Jean would remove the tumor.

Dr. Jean said he was going to do his best to preserve the facial nerve, which runs along the same area as the affected acoustic and vestibular nerves. If the tumor had attached itself firmly to the facial nerve, it would be difficult to remove it without doing a lot of damage. One of the options then would be to leave a little bit of tumor on the facial nerve in order to minimize the damage. Usually, that small bit of tumor would not grow once its blood flow was eliminated by the removal of the rest of the tumor. Otherwise, he would be forced to damage or cut the facial nerve in order to get all the tumor out. Cutting or severely damaging the facial nerve would leave me looking like a stroke victim permanently. I was obviously all in favor of preserving the facial nerve. I wasn't exactly a magazine advertising model or anything, but I wasn't a bad looking guy and I didn't really want a droopy face. There were a lot of things that went along with the "damaged or cut facial nerve" scenario that I didn't even really want to consider. There were discussions of putting a weight in my eyelid to help it close and things like that. I just ignored a lot of that information and acted like it wouldn't happen. I didn't know how else to handle it.

The last part of the surgery would be to remove a section of body fat from my abdomen (no need to worry about being able to find plenty of that!) and pack it into the hole in my skull to avoid any air gaps or abscesses that could occur. Then they would sew my ear flap back on and I'd be on my way to recovery. With all the cutting, drilling, filling, and stuff, it struck me as very similar to a weekend wood shop project. Even though this was obviously pretty involved, it seemed like losing the hearing in my left ear would be the worst of the long term effects of surgery as long as they were able to preserve the facial nerve.

Dr. Kim also asked me to go see an Ophthalmologist to be sure that the tumor wasn't affecting my optic nerve or any of the related visual systems. Yet another medical appointment. It was really starting to feel like that's all I did anymore was schedule and go to medical appointments. But I made an appointment with an Ophthalmologist in the town nearest us.

I usually used a different eye doctor office, but they did not have an Ophthalmologist on staff at the location I usually went to, so I went to another office. The two eye practices turned out to be across the highway from each other. The eye doctor took me through a barrage of tests to make sure that there wasn't any damage to my eyes or optic nerve. He even took pictures of the back of my eye and showed me where the optic nerve connection was made. At the end of a full afternoon of testing, he determined that the tumor was not adversely affecting my eye.

Just as a point of information- there are other surgical approaches that are used to gain access to these tumors. There was one in particular that entered the skull behind the ear that my surgical team was not in favor of because of the need to manipulate the brain to allow access to the tumor. This manipulation runs the risk of a permanent brain injury which can result in chronic debilitating headaches (or worse). There are plenty of success stories out there with these approaches as well. Again, I'm not a doctor, I'm just telling you what my experience was. It is just an important reminder of the need to discuss with any medical professional the possible good and bad side-effects and outcomes of different options. I did bump into a guy working as a salesman at a guitar shop one day whose wife had gone with one of the behind the ear surgical options and ended up with the chronic headaches. He said she faced a daily choice of horribly painful headaches and a clearly functioning mind, or using very strong pain killers to be comfortable and then deal with not being terribly coherent due to the drugs. I think I'll stick with losing the hearing in one ear if those are the alternatives.

You are probably also still feeling like this is some rare, almost never diagnosed brain tumor, right? You've never heard of Acoustic

Neuroma before? Or if you have, you've been told it's incredibly rare? The owner of that guitar store's wife also had an Acoustic Neuroma. The owner, the salesman, and I all stood around in the owner's office for a few minutes telling stories. Three random people, all standing in his office who had been affected by this "rare" thing. Don't forget the coworker of our friend, Rick. Oh, and Smitty's brother-in-law. And then there was... well, you get the idea. It isn't actually that rare, it's just not well publicized.

I couldn't decide if I was comforted by the fact that I wasn't alone in all of this, or if I was really angry that the initial diagnosis had been blundered so badly by that first nurse practitioner. I guess it was a little of both. I felt very alone, even though I had discovered that this type of tumor wasn't as rare as we had first thought. I'm sure that's how all newly diagnosed patients feel with any type of disease or problem. But you're not alone. Don't let yourself feel isolated. We're all in this thing together!

I was doing a lot of research (on our new laptop) at this point about Acoustic Neuroma. I read every online article, journal, discussion, etc... that I could find. The one thing that I didn't think to do was try to connect with other patients. I still thought of it as a rare condition, so I didn't bother to look. I would have found a substantial amount of information if I had thought to look for it. There is a stellar group on Facebook, users on Twitter, and several different discussion forums all providing a wealth of experiences of different people. These outlets provide people a place to share their experiences, support others, and learn about alternatives that they might not have been aware of. Obviously, none of these things should ever replace the advice of a doctor, but they are a valuable resource that I overlooked before my surgery. We've all seen what I did when I was given information about the surgery, though, so maybe my lack of engagement with other patients kindly saved me more fainting spells.

4 - PREPARATION

The time had come for me to start getting things ready for the surgery date. It was scheduled for Tuesday, July 21st, 2009. I had a couple of weeks to get all my ducks in a row. We had to start lining up things like somewhere for Bogey to go. Luckily, the greyhound community is very tight-knit, and there was another family near us that was happy to have Bogey come visit while I was going to be in the hospital. We also needed to find someone to help with the responsibilities involved in taking care of our vacation rental. Two things happened here that worked out really well. First, our renters for the time I was scheduled to be in the hospital were great. They were very patient when a tree fell in a windstorm. Second, Kay's brother, Brian, came out to visit and take care of my normal work responsibilities with our rental house.

I had a bit of a crisis of conscience a few days before the surgery. It's one I haven't really talked about since those nervous days before I went to the hospital. I have this theory that as a society we save too many people. But now it was my turn. How could I justify this to myself? If I were having my appendix out or something, it wouldn't have been a big deal. But how could I explain the fact that we were going to use the time, resources, and what would probably be tens or hundreds of thousands of dollars that could all be put to better use? This was a real ethical dilemma for me.

I was also afraid. Kay and I had put a happy face on all this, and would continue to do so, but on that Saturday, just three days before the surgery, I couldn't keep the smile on my face any longer. I couldn't even put my finger on what I was frightened of. I just knew I was scared. I wasn't really worried about not surviving the surgery since the doctors we had met were top notch. It was sort of like the fear that I imagine grips people who are sky diving for the first time. I don't think they are really nervous that the parachute won't open, since I would guess that is pretty rare. It's just the fear of the unknown. There wasn't anything for me to compare this experience with in my life up to that point. I was simply afraid. Having my fear and my ethics both hit me at once put me into a combative mood where I didn't want to have the surgery. It was a pretty dark place for me to be.

My wife and I had a very long conversation that day about both my ethical dilemma and my growing fear. I really did not want to go through with the surgery. You can imagine how frustrated Kay was. Her stubborn ass of a husband was going to skip having a surgery that could save him in favor of a certain decline into a vegetative state that she'd have to deal with before the tumor eventually killed him. These are moments when she often uses the phrase, "Hands off ladies, he's all mine." I don't blame her. It was a selfish thing for me to want. I just want to be clear here- I'm no saint. I have fears and unreasonable expectations just like anybody else. I'm pretty lucky that Kay is so understanding and patient with me. I know how angry I get about the little things in life. Heck, my heart-rate and blood pressure skyrocket when people drive too slow in the passing lane. I'm sure I would have been shaking and shouting about how stupid I was if I had been in her place with me acting this way.

This particular conversation kept going round and round. It all started in the kitchen and had its major escalation there. That's usually my favorite place to be when I'm arguing with Kay- I lean against the counter in front of the sink with my arms crossed while I'm digging in my heels in our disagreement. Or maybe I'm just acting like a heel, but I suppose it depends on your viewpoint. She can always tell when I've completely stopped listening to reason when I step over to get a Diet Coke out of the refrigerator and bring it back to Gould. "Gould" was what we called the safe spot in tag games when we were kids. You probably called it "base" or "safe", but there were no such simple solutions growing up in small town Minnesota. Gould is the perfect name for this spot in the kitchen, since most of the arguments I have from that spot are pretty childish.

After a while of me being on Gould and digging my heels in, Kay usually gets frustrated and gives up. I could tell she was heartbroken on this occasion. I continued to follow my usual formula at this point and left my safe spot to join her in the family room so that we could come to some compromise. I was so scared to go through with the surgery. We were talking about brain surgery here. They were going to be poking around in my skull! What if they couldn't save my facial nerve? I don't want to sound too flippant or shallow, but I really wasn't interested in having half of my face not work for the rest of my life. I'd rather take my chances with the tumor than deal with the social stigmata of looking like a stroke victim for the next forty or fifty years.

I'm pretty sure that my wife understood my fear, but she was more afraid of what would happen to me if I didn't have the surgery than what could go wrong if I did. This was one of those "I love you no-matter what" moments for her. I think she just didn't want to lose me. Wow, no pressure there at all. I'll just go ahead and explain to my wonderful wife that I'd rather let the tumor kill me than have a flaccid face, while she breaks down in tears and explains that she'll love me however I look. Now I feel terrible. But this isn't just about her feelings about the matter. I would have to deal with going out in public like that every day. I'm sure I'd become a hermit. I'd just lock myself away somewhere and never come out. Am I really so shallow as all that? If I want to be honest with myself, the answer is an unequivocal: yes. There was something good that came out of all of this. I knew my wife had my back if I decided to go through with the surgery. That meant the world to me. No matter how alone I might feel, I could count on her to be there.

I finally decided to have the surgery done. What would finally sway me to change my mind and make me decide to go ahead with it? What incredible motivation or insight could make me see the light? More fear. I was terrified that, with the tumor pushing on my brain stem, I would end up a vegetable and somebody would make me live that way. We have all read about things like that happening in the news. I had this horrible scenario playing out in my head where I'd be brain dead and someone would figure out a way to go against my wishes because I hadn't expressed them clearly enough and I'd end up in some institution somewhere. They'd have me propped up in an iron-framed bed in striped pajamas and a towel under my chin to catch the drool. I'd have visitors once in a while for the first year or so, then I'd just lie there and drool until somebody forgot about me and the state finally decided that I wasn't worth the money to keep around. The fear of that scenario quickly over-ran any ethics I had and even overshadowed my fear of the brain surgery. The fear of having my face permanently screwed up was nothing in comparison to the sheer terror that came over me with the possibility of a scenario like that. And the face issue was far less likely than the drooling on my pj's option. I'll pick the less scary option every time. I am not ashamed to say that I am a complete and utter coward. The only thing needed to get me to put all those other things on a shelf was a deeper seated fear. But I was a coward who was going to have brain surgery on Tuesday, so maybe I was a brave coward.

I had started riding a bicycle for fun and exercise a little bit the previous summer and was really beginning to get interested in biking before my summer was interrupted with that whole brain tumor thing. Everybody knew that I wasn't going to be in any shape to ride much outside after the surgery, so my sister, her boyfriend, and my parents all chipped in on a nice CycleOps stationary bicycle trainer for me to use after the surgery to help me get my strength back. Mounting the rear wheel of my bike in the trainer would turn my bike into a stationary resistance trainer. I thought it was a great gift idea, since I'd be able to get back on my bike sooner by being in a safe, indoor environment rather than out on the roads alone.

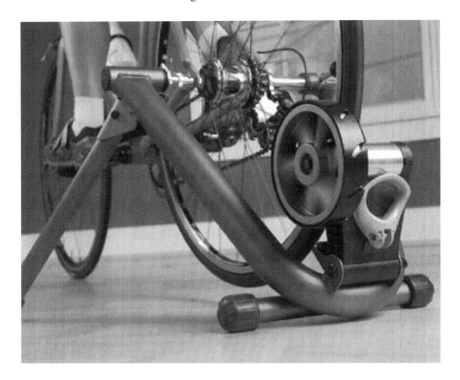

I mentioned before that my wife and I race on sailboats for fun. July 19-21 was the big local regatta for our region of the Chesapeake Bay. I chose not to do any racing since I knew that I'd be a basket case trying to get everything ready for the big day, but that didn't mean I couldn't hang out at the party! If you've never been to a sailing party, you are missing out. They are a huge social event with great music, lots of cold drinks, and a chance to see sailing friends you haven't seen in a while. I had strict instructions to consume no alcohol for at least twenty-four hours before my surgery along with the usual food and water cut-off times leading up to the procedure. When all my sailor friends saw me at the party on Sunday, they were stunned. "Aren't you having brain surgery?" they asked. Not 'til Tuesday, dammit! It was my opinion that, in the very unlikely event of something going horribly wrong on Tuesday, I wanted everyone's last memories of me to be of all of us having fun together. I even went to the party for a short visit on Monday afternoon (obviously not drinking). I wanted to be with my friends and loved ones. A lot of these people are close to me like family from all the time we had spent sailing together over the years.

If I'm honest, I'll also admit that I was a bit of an attention hound with my surgery so close. I think a lot of that is subconscious, but that doesn't make it less true. It's just part of my personality. There are people who will go through their entire birthday every year and not tell people. I'm not like that at all. I tell complete strangers that it's my birthday and then look at them expectantly for some sort of well wishes. I was the same way with the lead up to my surgery. You couldn't have gotten within a two block radius of me without knowing that I was having brain surgery on Tuesday.

I'm sure there are people who would be aghast at the idea of me spending what could possibly be my last couple of days on earth partying with my friends, but when it comes down to a situation like the one I was presented with, I think you just have to do what is right for you. Besides, I was with my wife. I'm not a religious person, so there wasn't much point in trying to save my soul. Let's be honest here- I'm going to hell in three languages, and I'm working on Latvian. I just couldn't think of anywhere I would rather be than drinking rum with my friends at a sailing party. Obviously other people would need to figure out where that place would be for them. Hopefully they would spend it playing catch with their kids, or reading to their grandchildren, or playing ping-pong if the desire was there. It doesn't matter to me what you do. I figure it's the right thing if you say so, just make sure it's what you want to do and doesn't step on other people. I'm not really a pessimist, but there's no way to know what's going to happen on that surgical table. Why not make sure your last couple of days prior to surgery are spent right? I don't expect people who haven't been placed in this situation to understand. Maybe they'll just take my word for it. I hope that none of them are ever put in a situation where they have to make that decision in their own life.

Kay and I put on our happy faces and did our best to have a "devil may care" attitude about the whole thing. Even though we had the conversation about whether or not I wanted to go ahead with the surgery, that really seemed a distant memory; a bump in the road. Other than that one conversation, neither of us had really allowed ourselves to think much about the severity of the situation. Everything in our situation had gone back to feeling like it was happening around us rather than happening to us. We had become spectators in our own lives again. We kept telling ourselves and others that "it was going to be what it was going to be." Right. Good plan. Keep it lighthearted and we'll be fine... Yeah, hang on a bit and we'll see how that works out.

On Monday night I finished packing up the few things I had been told to bring with me to the hospital and laid out the clothes I was going to wear in the morning. What do you bring along to brain surgery? To be honest, not much. The hospital had been pretty specific about me bringing a loose fitting set of clothes to wear when I got discharged. They were even kind enough to remind me to make sure it was a button-down shirt so I wouldn't have to drag any kind of pull-over across my incision site. I brought my toiletries kit, and even a paperback book- though I wouldn't ever read a page of it. So basically, I just had a little ditty bag.

Kay brought a journal style notebook to keep track of what was happening and have an easy place to keep notes on any instructions the medical staff might have. She also brought along our new laptop to make updating everyone a little easier. Social media hadn't taken over yet, so she planned to use email and a specialty site, www.caringbridge.org, that Georgetown had suggested.

In today's world of Facebook, Twitter, Google Plus, and countless other social media outlets, you'd think there was no need for a specialty medical communication site like CaringBridge. I think you'd be mistaken. CaringBridge offers people a unique way to keep in touch with loved ones by posting updates to their CaringBridge page, then loved ones can post messages back in the guest book. This format allows a family to concentrate on getting better while still keeping everyone informed, but not having to send out countless emails or make hours worth of phone calls. It also keeps family and friends from all over the world connected during the patient's journey. If you aren't familiar with them, take a jaunt over to their website at www.caringbridge.org. Maybe make a donation to help them with their mission to help make health journeys easier for families. I'd also suggest using them if the need arises in your future!

Then it was the big day: Tuesday, July 21st 2009. With the ninety minute drive to Georgetown and the 5:30am arrival time, morning came very quickly. The car ride into town was uneventful since even Washington, DC traffic isn't bad at 4:00am. There was an understandable nervous tension in the car. I don't remember what

Kay and I talked about, but it evidently wasn't earth-shattering. We arrived a little early since the drive had been so simple. We kept ourselves busy with a short pre-dawn walk and even a "before" picture. I now hate that picture for so many reasons, but we'll discuss those later.

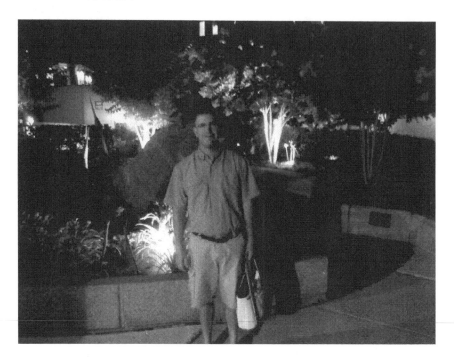

The surgery center opened up and we went in and got registered. Our nurse, Alma, took us back into the prep area. Kay was allowed back with me, which was really nice. I don't think I would have done very well alone. I'm sure I would have had at least one panic attack, given how nervous I was. The prep area was set up with curtains around wheeled gurneys so multiple patients could be getting ready at the same time. Being so early, they didn't have many lights on yet. It seemed like they just had a few curtained sections lit for the early arrivals. It reminded me of getting to the pet supply store right after they open. A "In an effort to be more environmentally conscious, we use half lighting until 10:00am" sort of thing. We were the first ones back there, so there was still some humor while changing into my gown and the socks with the gripper things on the bottoms, including some fun discussion of the very stylish icky tan color of my grippy socks. Another teenage patient and her Mom came into the prep area one curtain over from us a few minutes later. On their side, there was a lot of nervous talk, tears, and hugs & kisses. Still sticking with the humor in our prep area, we chuckled at the drama over there given the difference between the two surgeries about to happen. The girl was having her tonsils taken out, while I was having brain surgery. Don't get me wrong here, I'm not trying to diminish the risk involved in her procedure at all. We just found it funny at the time given our efforts to keep things lighthearted. I wonder what the family of the girl having her tonsils out thought was going on with me given all the laughs.

Next came all the details of the surgical prep. Several nurses came in to see me and asked me to confirm my name and personal information and what procedure I was having done, then have me sign the confirmation documents. My IV was inserted, thankfully without any panicky incidents on my part. After that I felt like an elderly royal holding court. I was propped up on my gurney, snuggled comfortably in a warm blanket while a procession of people was brought to me. Being a University Hospital, there were a lot of medical students that came in to examine me. They were all very nice, and I was glad to be able to help provide some good information for their medical studies. During their examinations of me, each of them would hold my face in their hands and rub their thumbs lightly along my cheeks under my eyes. "Can you feel that?" Yep. All the doctors and students were still surprised that the tumor hadn't done any obvious damage to my facial nerve up to this point. Some of them were so surprised after seeing the MRI images that they seemed like they didn't believe me when I told them that I could feel their thumb rubbing my cheek just fine. I hoped that my case was one that the students could file away for the future and be more informed professionals having had the experience.

Both of my doctors came in to talk to me and to confirm which side they were doing surgery on. They even marked me with a marker on my left ear to confirm which side was being operated on. It was funny to me that the marker was sealed in plastic and had to be unwrapped before they drew the mark on my ear. I guess the rules for cleanliness are really strict; otherwise I would have offered to loan them the marker in the trunk of Kay's Volvo. I was really impressed with the level of care taken to make sure that there were no mistakes made. Even though I knew I was in a top medical facility with excellent doctors, I was still nervous. Their level of professional preparation did a lot to boost my confidence about what was next. I kept the humor and nonchalance level up by asking Dr. Kim if he could sew my ear back on level with the other one. My left ear, the one being operated on, was naturally just a little lower than my right. He looked at me like I was an alien. Like I had no idea how serious the surgery that was about to happen to me was. I couldn't help it; humor was the only defense mechanism that was working. We just weren't allowing ourselves to think about the seriousness that Dr. Kim obviously took for granted. He did nod and smile at me as he left.

Finally, it was time for the anesthesiologist to come in to talk to me and start getting me hooked up to his equipment. Kay asked him about whether or not I might be restrained after a conversation that we had with a friend of ours who had woken up from a long surgery to find that his hands had been tied firmly to the bed. The anesthesiologist seemed to think we were nuts. No, there wouldn't be any need for restraints. Whew! I was glad to hear it. Waking up tied to the bed didn't sound like fun at all.

He and some of the nurses were the latest in the list of people surprised by our happy attitude and nonchalance. They instructed my wife and I to go ahead and say goodbye for the day and we'd see each other after the surgery. We made eye contact and all the happy-go-lucky went straight out the window. Kay has never been very good at concealing her emotions. She's very much a WYSIWYG (what you see is what you get) person. She was holding my hand and I looked over to her to say something funny. I saw her lip curl and a tear run down her cheek. Both of us completely lost it. All the emotion that we had been ignoring for the past couple of weeks came rushing out in a flurry of tears and realizations. This was serious business! I wasn't having my tonsils out, or my appendix, or something simple... I was having a large brain tumor removed. The Anesthesiologist gave us a moment or two until we were both in tears and blubbering incoherently, then all went black.

Part 2 - Surgery

5 - INTROSPECTION

"I learned that courage was not the absence of fear, but the triumph over it. The brave man is not he who does not feel afraid, but he who conquers that fear." - Nelson Mandella

Up to this point, my story has been all about facts and events. I chased around a diagnosis that was very hard to pinpoint. I wasted a year ignoring the ever worsening symptoms. I found the right doctors to diagnose and develop a plan of action to deal with my tumor. I have shared some of the hard discussions about even harder decisions. I have even tried to prepare for something I wasn't emotionally equipped to deal with. There were a lot of superfluous television references and some bad jokes. But those were all just things that happened. They were the facts of the situation, which culminated in me being put under for surgery. I have talked in depth about those facts, now let's talk about the truth.

My wife and I had been living out our happy little existence. We were sailing, both figuratively and literally, though life. She was the problem solver, the bread winner, the responsible one, and obviously the left-brain. I was the artist, the musician, the free thinker, the idea guy, the right-brain. You couldn't make a better pair if you were writing nursery rhymes. We were Jack Sprat and his wife for the Twenty-first Century. Then along came a spider- OK, it was a tumor, but try to work with the nursery rhyme theme for me. It sat down in my head and ruined everything.

Sudden hardship is nothing new in life, it has been part of the human condition throughout history, and we deal with it all the time. People we know get sick, or they struggle with things, and they die.

Such is the nature of life. Until it happens to you. Not a friend, a co-worker, or even an immediate family member, but you.

There is even an amazing spirit in most people that wishes that they could take on the burdens of others. A parent wishing it was they in the car accident instead of their child. A person wishing it was their cancer diagnosis instead of it happening to their spouse. A buddy wishing he was the one in the line of fire instead of his friend. Those are such strong and generous desires, but it doesn't work that way.

When I finally got the answer to the questions about my symptoms, I was overcome. If some hero had suddenly appeared to push me out of the way of the locomotive that was my brain tumor, I would have been thrilled. If there was any way that I could have traded it to you and your desire to help carry my burden, that tumor would have been yours. In a heartbeat. That sounds selfish. Yes, it is. I was terrified. I was angry. I was frustrated. I was distraught, and I was about to become unglued.

How had this happened to me? What on earth had I ever done to deserve this? I find myself wanting to write bad jokes here. I guess that's because there aren't any answers to those questions. The jokes aren't going to help find things that don't exist. Finally, I guess I realized that everybody who deals with even the slightest hardship asks these questions, but I didn't really care. This was my hardship. I had a brain tumor.

There's no way to describe the terror involved. I can tell you I was afraid. I could even try to creatively compare it to something to give you the feeling of being in my situation. I could tell you it was like staring down the barrel of a gun in an effort to describe the trembling fear I felt. I could compare it to being lost at sea or stranded on a desert island to convey the complete isolation I felt. But, while those analogies might give you a concept of the feelings, they would never come close enough to representing the true nature of how I felt. I don't think enough empathy exists to ever give those feelings justice in someone that hasn't had the experience.

I'm not the "I'm going to fight this. It's not going to get the best of me!" type of person. I hear descriptions of people who have lost "battles" with disease all the time. There was no fighting a brain tumor. The fact that it was there meant I had already lost any "battle" there might have been long before I even realized I was supposed to fight. I guess that warrior mentality must help other people deal with their hardship. Whatever works for them is all right by me, but that just isn't how I approach things like this.

As much as I didn't see a way to fight the tumor, I did come close to giving up when I found myself too frightened to have the surgery. Why couldn't there be a way that I could fix it? Why couldn't there be a way that I could do something to make it better? Some diet or exercise program, or a medication that I could take. But it wasn't going to be like that. I felt so much like giving up. I guess that must be why people fight; the only other alternative is surrender. The feeling of that surrender is a scary thing. It's such a lonely place. That's the bottom of a hole I hope I never see again in my life. Had it been just a couple of inches deeper, it would have ended by my hand. The option of having the doctors try to get it out was the couple of inches I needed. But even the surgery keeping me those couple of inches off the bottom of the hole was terrifying. They were going to cut off my ear and drill a hole in my head!

How did I deal with my fear? I didn't deal with it, not really. I was just scared. I was scared of the concept of having a tumor growing in my head, pushing on stuff. I was scared out of my wits at the thought of having somebody drill a hole in my head. Hell, I passed out when the doctor told me they were going to cut off my ear- I never even got to the drilling part.

But the quote from Nelson Mandella talked about triumphing over fear, conquering it. Conquer, I could do. How? When I was first faced with my diagnosis and all the gritty details that went along with it, the fear overwhelmed me. I passed out. I freaked out. I flipped out. I quickly realized that I wouldn't be able to function if I tried to face it all at once, so I compartmentalized the fear. I conquered one part at a time.

The first time I really felt overwhelmed by my situation was obviously the diagnosis that I got from Dr. Marinelli: You've got a brain tumor. Everything else in the world stopped at that moment. That's how I deal with things like this. My entire world revolved around that one statement that he made in his office on that Tuesday morning while I was staring at that giant white lump in my head on that MRI scan. If you had asked me about anything else in my life at that point, my answer would have been given with a blank stare, "I have a brain tumor." What did I have for lunch today? "I have a brain tumor." That fear got sealed up tight in its own little box.

From there, I allowed myself to let little bits and pieces of my life back in. I need to tell my wife. I need to tell my family. I have to figure out what I'm going to do. I need to start working on getting this fixed. I didn't allow myself to think too far ahead yet. That was a bridge too far at that point.

That got me through to my appointment with Dr. Kim when he told me they were going to cut my ear off. We're not even talking about compartmentalizing fear anymore; we're talking about abject terror. It was that classic moment of all-consuming fear that causes people to stand and watch as the giant wave washes over them. I just got swept away. I was staring out the window in the airplane, calm and quiet as you please, while I watched the ground race towards me in a sickening spiral. How do you compartmentalize a statement from your doctor that makes you pass out? Very carefully. There wasn't even room for all the fear I had already been working with, so all that had to go. We'll just bury that box of fear in the back yard for now and dig it up when we have time to sort through it. Now for that whole ear cutting thing: take a deep breath, hold Kay's hand, hold it a little tighter, look Dr. Kim in the eye- and let's move forward. Alright, you're going to cut off my ear. Then what? I had to hold on to this one for a while. I couldn't be bothered with being afraid of having a hole drilled in my head or even the actual process of having the tumor cut out. We were going to just have to stick with the part about cutting off my ear. When I say that fear was all consuming, I mean it. You could have covered me with venomous snakes and all I would have been thinking about was my box that held the fear of having my ear cut off. There wasn't anything you could say or do that would make me loosen my vice-like grip holding that lid closed.

Under all of the other fears was the little gremlin of the potential for my face to be deformed for the rest of my life. That particular fear I left in the best compartment of all: the external one. I didn't internalize that fear since I didn't think that I'd be able to cope. So I did the next best thing- I ignored it. It still reared up and scared the pants off me once in a while, but I was able to keep it at bay for the most part. I think it was a lot like the myth about beating a lie detector test. The story goes that if you can convince yourself that your lie is actually the truth, you can beat a polygraph. True? It doesn't really matter. I had convinced myself that the possibility of having my facial nerve damaged to the point of deformity just didn't exist. I just went through my day and tried to never let that fear enter my mind. Was it the best solution, or the one that a psychologist would suggest? Probably not. It seems like something that a child would come up with. I guess that makes sense given the fact that I spent half of my MRI singing songs to my dancing toes. But it got me through, and that was all that really mattered.

The physical act of surgery was harder to sequester. Lying on the gurney in the surgical prep area left me very little wiggle room to work around the fact that I was about to have surgery. The medical students coming in to examine me and get a look at a patient that miraculously still had use of his face was a wake-up call. And all the jokes in the world weren't going to mask the obvious things like the gown I was wearing, the IV sticking out of my arm, the doctors & nurses coming and going, and those ridiculously ugly socks with the rubber grips on the bottoms. So that compartment wasn't sealed very well and leaked fear in the form of a flood of tears down my cheeks when I saw my wife start to cry. Luckily for me, the anesthesiologist was well armed with a whole barrage of fear container sealant and took care of it for me. His anesthesia meds were the best caulking I ever could have asked for to seal up my leaking box of fear.

The compartmentalization method may not have been the best coping mechanism to work with my fears, but it was all I could come up with. I wasn't offered any counseling. Compartmentalizing did manage to get me through the day. All I had to tell myself was that we needed to make it through to the end of each day and we would have succeeded. I could worry about tomorrow when I woke up. Just keep each fear sealed as tightly in its box as we can until I go to sleep, and things will be all right. That was true. It was, however, not much fun. Spending a couple of weeks trying to contain my fear while I ran around getting things set up so that I could be out of commission for a while was really stressful. I got myself wound up so tight a couple of times that I snapped. Luckily, when I snapped, it mostly just involved me being really depressed for an afternoon. After that little bit of downtime, I could get myself back to being afraid.

6 – KAY'S PERSPECTIVE

Obviously I wasn't awake or aware during the surgery, so what follows in this section is taken from my wife's journal that she kept through the day of July 21st and a day or two after, along with some recollections and some bits and pieces that I've picked up along the way. Most of these events will get repeated at some point when I relate the same time period from my perspective. I would like to start with the documented version of what actually happened, though, since I think it will be a good benchmark for comparison with my recollection later on. Please keep in mind that things will seem kind of dry throughout this section since my wife is a very fact-oriented, type "A" personality.

After the anesthesiologist juiced me and everything went black, I was taken to the operating room at about 7:45am. The surgery started officially at 8:41am. I have seen pictures of what I assume to be a similar device to the clamp that my head and shoulders were placed in to facilitate the surgery. Obviously, I needed to have my head and body completely immobilized. There are also all sorts of other things they do in final preparation for the surgery, some of which I would discover later. I saw footage of a man being prepped for brain surgery on a television documentary. They had him all hooked into the head clamp. I had to turn the channel. Even years later, I'm not sure I'd be able to watch that. To me, that clamp is like what a bone saw must have been like to a Civil War soldier. Seeing it gave me chills, knowing that it was the device that held me in place while the surgery was happening. It was the tool that made everything possible. It's definitely something that I would run away from if I ever saw it in a display of medical devices in a science museum. I'll try to avoid screaming hysterically while running away- should that situation ever come up.

Kay went to the surgical waiting area where she met her sister, Marcia, who had come to offer emotional support while I was in surgery. Kay evidently spent the first hour or so in tears, still gripped by the emotional outburst that we had down in the prep area. I suppose I should consider myself lucky that my most stressful moments were past while some of Kay's most nerve-wracking hours were just beginning. If something bad happened to me during the surgery, I wouldn't even notice. My wife would be the one that would have to cope with the loss.

Kay was given updates at 9:45am and 11:30am that everything was going fine. Dr. Kim was in surgery with me at that point working on the entry process. He finished the first part of the surgery at about 1:00pm, when Dr. Jean began the Neurosurgery part of the procedure. At this point, I was still stable and everything was going as planned.

What was Kay doing during all this time, you might ask? Sitting. Worrying. She had been able to get herself past the initial emotions of the day and had stopped crying. She was trying to keep everyone up to date via email with the information she was being given. Luckily, Kay had a lot of support just like I did. Kay's sister stayed all day and into the night to sit with her, and she got a nice visit from our friend, Peter. She was very thankful to have friends and family to be there to support her.

There were a lot of people supporting me through all of this, with Kay obviously being the key support person. But who supports the supporters? Who offers reassurance and support to the one person who has to bear the burden of keeping a smile on her face and standing tall so that I can lean on her? Family and friends. I cannot stress enough how important these people were up to this point and for many months to come. Imagine how terrible and lonely it would have been for Kay to come out of the surgical prep area in tears and spend the rest of the day alone. Having her sister there to comfort her and help her work through the emotions of the day was very important. Having someone to listen to all of the feelings and fears that had previously been bottled up inside and were now pouring out in a tearful jumble.

There were other people who had volunteered to be available to us for support as well. My parents and brother had offered to come to town for support, but we politely suggested they stay home. We knew how stressful things would be during the time around the surgery, and having company from out of town that didn't know the ins and outs of Washington, DC traffic would just create even more stress. They were very understanding about it.

At about 6:30pm, Dr. Kim rejoined Dr. Jean in surgery as they prepared for the final part of the procedure and getting everything sewn back up and bandaged. Dr. Jean came out to talk to Kay at about 8:45pm to give her another update. He told her that the surgery had gone well and that Dr. Kim was working to finish things up and that I would probably be in surgery until about 10:00pm. He said that the tumor had been attached pretty firmly to both my facial nerve and my brain stem. They had been able to successfully dislodge the tumor from my brain stem, but they couldn't fully remove the tumor from my facial nerve without causing a lot of damage. At that point, Dr. Jean decided to leave a small sliver of the tumor attached to the facial nerve. He said that the facial nerve should be OK after some temporary weakness from the disturbance and that the tumor should not grow again now that they had cut off its blood flow by removing the main part of the tumor. Whew!

The doctors had sent the tumor out for pathology just to confirm that it was indeed an Acoustic Neuroma and that it was not malignant. They were going to keep me intubated overnight so that they could keep me under observation to be sure that there were no issues.

One of my favorite stories from this particular part of the process happened during this last conversation between Kay and Dr. Jean. When Dr. Jean told my wife that he had been able to preserve the integrity of the facial nerve by leaving the tiny slice of tumor attached to it, she replied that I would be relieved since that was one of my biggest worries about all this. Dr. Jean replied that the surgical team's worries usually focused more around making sure that nothing went wrong that could endanger the safety of their patient. This really struck me as funny later on when she told me about it. I was more worried about my "beautiful" face, while Dr.

Jean and the surgical team were busy making sure that I didn't end up with a brain injury or dead. I never even would have thought of that. I guess I just left the finer points up to the doctors. Me considering "dead" a finer point that the doctors were worried about is such a great example of the fear that I had compartmentalized. I knew that there was no way that I would ever be able to work through the fear that would come with the possibility that I might not survive the surgery. I didn't even bother to consider it; I just put it in a box and shoved in in the very darkest back corner of the closet.

It also shows the level of trust that had been developed between myself and both surgeons. Once I had found a good team to take care of my little tumor friend, all that fear could just go in the box and go away. Like I said before, I wouldn't even notice if things all went horribly wrong. What did I care?

At about 10:15pm, Dr. Kim came out and told Kay that they had finished the surgery and would be taking me to the Neuro Intensive Care Unit, which they did at about 11:00pm.

7 – THE NEURO ICU

The surgery had lasted about fourteen hours. It was complete and Dr. Kim and Dr. Jean had gotten the tumor out. But things were far from over.

At about midnight they did some basic testing to be sure I was still in there after being in surgery for so long. They checked for responses in my eyes, hands, and feet. I was evidently agitated when they were doing these tests, so they started me on a Propofol drip to try to keep me calm and help me sleep. They followed this up at 12:15am with Fentanyl via my IV for pain and to keep my blood pressure down. Fentanyl is a narcotic that is about one hundred times more powerful than morphine. At least they weren't skimping on the good stuff, right? At 12:20am I was x-rayed again to confirm the position of my breathing tube and a blood pressure specific medication was added to my IV mix to try to lower my blood pressure below 160 from the 170's it was in. They continued to monitor my condition throughout the night and tested my eyes, hands, and feet for response hourly.

It's a little weird for me to think that I had a machine helping me breathe and that people were checking to make sure I was still "in there." The worst medical thing that had ever happened to me before this was a really badly skinned knee incident that happened on the second date my wife and I went on. We were rollerblading and I had been showing off. The nurse in the emergency room had threatened to make me clean out my own knee with the brush. And then there had been the broken toe on the boat, but nothing that had ever involved me needing a machine to help me breathe. It still makes me shake my head a little bit to realize what an involved surgery this had been. I feel bad when I hear on the news that someone was in a car accident and was in surgery for eight hours. But there's also a part of me now that says, "Meh. Eight hours? That's not so bad." I know, I'm not the nicest person in the world when I feel that way, but thanks for pointing it out anyway. I do really feel bad for people who have to have multiple surgeries in a short amount of time. I don't ever want anything to do with that.

I'm going to keep on with Kay's notes and the actual account of what happened when I woke up that morning. I think it will help give some reference for my later description of the same events from my viewpoint when I woke up. I'm pretty sure it will also show just how much effect the anesthesia and drugs had in clouding my perception and understanding of things, how much it altered my view of the passage of time, and how it affected my feelings and mood. It's also just very entertaining to compare the two.

It was about 8:00am when I started to wake up. I had been unconscious, anesthetized, and then sedated and given powerful pain medications for just over twenty-four hours. When I woke, Kay's journal describes me as being "somewhat agitated" and complaining of being hot. My ICU nurse, Kristina, kindly put some ice packs around me to help me cool off. They had put pneumatic massage sleeves on my lower legs to help my blood circulation. They seemed to be too tight and were making me uncomfortable, so the nurse loosened them. The nurses had, in order to keep me from disturbing my breathing tube, placed my wrists in medical restraints. I reacted very badly to this, but they loosened them and got me to calm down.

We used paper and pen to communicate, since I still had the breathing tube inserted. Kay's notes suggest that I had been unhappy with someone and had some pretty nasty descriptives for them. I also asked what day it was. My reaction to hearing it was only Wednesday, one day after the surgery, seemed "deflated." It seemed as if I wished it was further along in the recovery process and maybe a little closer to going home. Unfortunately, it was only the first day. Going home was still a long way off in the future.

Once the nurses and Kay helped me get a little more comfortable and calmed down, my demeanor grew more positive along with the written questions I was asking. I asked about what happened in the Tour de France while I was out. I was also very happy to hear about all the well wishes from friends and family. I have to admit that I am glad that the strangest thing I was asking about here was the bike race. I think there was an opportunity there for me to ask some really embarrassing questions. Hurray for my brain having its filters on even when I was all drugged up!

At about 9:00am, the nurse increased my sedative in order to keep me a little more calm and help me rest. She also changed the mixture being pumped into my breathing tube to test how close I was getting to being able to breathe on my own. They kept that mixture for about thirty minutes to see what the result would be. The test seemed successful, so they kept me on the reduced mixture. Nurse Kristina then administered some medications including some normal medications that I take each morning, something to help protect my stomach, a stool softener, and some insulin to help keep my blood sugar levels correct. The physician's assistant on duty returned and said that further study of the breathing tests showed that the fluid levels were a little off, so they increased fluid levels in my mixture again. And finally, at 11:30am, my breathing tube was taken out. They kept an oxygen line connected to my nose.

The amount of care, concern, and attention that was being paid to me says a lot for my condition during the first hours of my surgical recovery. I was awake, stable, and whole- but there was still a lot of work and detail that needed to be attended to. They helped me turn onto my side and rest, at which point Kay went to get a bite to eat for lunch.

I continued to rest most of the afternoon. Dr. Jean stopped in during the afternoon to check on me and chatted a little. He told us how well he thought the surgery had gone. A resident from Dr. Kim's team also stopped by to check on me. Kay asked him about how often the dressing and bandage on my surgical site would be changed. He said that it would probably be changed on Thursday or Friday and that Dr. Kim would be in on Thursday and we could follow up with him then.

At around 5:00pm, Nurse Kristina tried to administer some more medication in pill form. I took each pill with a little water but vomited them back up, along with everything else that had been in my stomach. Mostly all over Nurse Kristina. Oops. Even though I hadn't felt dizzy or nauseous before or after my vomiting spell, it was decided that we should probably skip my evening meal since I obviously wasn't quite up to having things in my stomach yet. They went ahead and removed the oxygen line from my nose at this point. I slept after that for a couple of hours. Kay made note that it was the best sleep I had gotten since that morning without the help of additional sedation.

Later that evening, around 10:00pm, we tried the medication again. It seemed to stay down this time. Though about a half-hour later, I was starting to feel nauseous again so they administered some Zofran (an anti-nausea medication) into my IV to help calm down my queasiness. Then I got some more sleep.

The next morning was Thursday, now twenty-four hours since I woke up and had begun my recovery. At about 8:00am I had a little bit of warm chicken broth, three pieces of Jello, and a little bit of grape juice along with some water.

At about 10:30am, Nurse Kristina came in with my morning pills. This time it included a potassium pill in addition to my regular daily medications. First she gave me a little applesauce, then I tried half of the potassium pill. Yes, actually, you guessed right! I vomited my breakfast all over her again. A little while later they administered some Zofran through my IV again to try to help my stomach feel better. You could tell at this point that Nurse Kristina was even less thrilled with me barfing all over her than I was. And I wasn't much thrilled being sick again.

We tried my regular pills again around noon. I managed to get one pill down without incident. Then they brought me a little bit of lunch: beef broth, Jello, applesauce, and some cherry ice. I also had a little ginger ale and apple juice. They decided not to push their luck by trying to get me to take the potassium or a steroid orally. Those went into my IV instead. I got some more rest after lunch.

I find the things that my wife took notes on fascinating. The complete menu for each of my meals is a little bit of overkill in my opinion. I understand her desire to be sure I was getting enough caloric intake, but writing down that I ate three clumps of Jello rather than just "some" is funny. But I guess I can't complain since without her notes we'd be stuck with just my recollections. And while those won't be as boring, they certainly aren't going to be this accurate, either.

They stepped down my status from being an ICU/Critical Care patient at about 4:45pm. This meant that they could remove all the heart monitors and an arterial line, which had been keeping a constant check on my blood pressure. They did leave my Foley catheter, my IV, plus my back-up IV in place.

This brings us to a good time to talk about what family and loved ones should be ready for if they are going to be there for the immediate recovery of any patient who has undergone a major surgical procedure like mine. There is going to be a lot of apparatus and paraphernalia hooked up to the patient. You can expect to see tubes and wires and all manner of complicated looking stuff poking out from their body. I think it could be very overwhelming to a loved one who was not expecting to see the patient hooked to it all. We were lucky to have had a friend warn Kay about the probability of me being hooked to all sorts of stuff, so she wasn't put off by it. And Kay is usually very businesslike about things like that, just so long as there wasn't a spider anywhere to be seen. Then all bets are off. It seems like medical professionals are concentrating so hard on making sure their patients are getting the best care possible, that they might forget sometimes about the shock that the invasive nature of medicine can have on regular people. They don't warn the patient, either. We'll see an embarrassingly extreme example of that when we read about my reaction to all this stuff.

Since I was no longer in a critical or ICU status, I was moved to a regular room in the neurology ward later that evening.

I would like to take just a minute to offer a thought or two on nurses. Even though I did my best to be a polite and cooperative patient, Nurse Kristina and other members of the staff went through a lot of difficulty with me. She dealt with me during my struggles and uncooperative behavior when I woke up on Wednesday morning. She even got vomited on a couple of times! Yet she was always polite, upbeat, and very professional at every turn with Kay and me. I don't understand at all how nurses can be barfed on multiple times and still have a smile on their face the next time they come in the room. I know I couldn't do it. I can't ever thank Nurse Kristina or the thousands of nurses everywhere just like her enough. I certainly gained a healthy new respect for them and the things they do. And I promise that I'll do my best not to puke on them anymore.

8 – MY PERSPECTIVE

Now that we've had a chance to go through the real time-line of events as they actually happened, I can relate to you my point of view of those same events. Keep in mind that I was still working through the effects of the anesthesia, and was on some very potent pain medications, sedatives, and even stool softeners. I have no recollection of anything that took place on Tuesday night after the surgery, so my story begins when I woke up on Wednesday morning.

Noise. Lots of jumbled noise. I hear a voice. I think someone is calling my name. Why do they keep calling my name? "Chris? Can you hear me, Chris?" *Where the hell am I? I try to answer, but I can't. Something is really wrong. Why can't I talk? Why can't I see? Where the hell am I?! All that noise. What is all that noise? And who keeps calling my name?*

Do you remember the movie version of Dalton Trumbo's "Johnny Got His Gun" from the 1970's? And the black and white sequences of Johnny panicking and thrashing when he can't see or tell what's happening to him? He's got the oddly shaped white cone covering his face. It didn't look like much fun, that's for sure. But that's about the only thing I can compare to that morning when I woke up. As surreal as it sounds, I couldn't communicate with anyone around me, but I was having a similar style of one-sided conversation as Johnny had in my head. Thankfully, I wasn't wondering why they were cutting off my arm or my leg, but there were a lot of other things going through my mind like *Why can't I see? What's wrong with my eyes? Did something bad happen to my eyes?*

I slowly started to discover things. I still couldn't figure out why I couldn't see, but realized that I couldn't answer whoever was calling my name because there was something (my breathing tube) shoved down my throat. I must have reached for it or something, because they grabbed my arms and pinned them down. I struggled. I was put in hospital restraints- do you remember when they said that wouldn't happen? Yeah, well. Too bad. I was terrified. *You said you wouldn't do that. Don't tie me up! That's scaring me!* I was thrashing around on the gurney. *Where is Kay? She'll get them to untie me.*

Keep in mind that I've been out for over twenty-four hours at this point. I'm finally awake, but feeling very isolated due to being blind, mute, and now bound tight. I began to struggle more, but they got me calmed down after a couple of minutes to the point where they could communicate with me. *Please untie me, I can be good. I'll be good, I promise! Just please untie me- I'm really frightened.*

Somewhere in life I learned to finger-spell in American Sign Language. Don't ask me where. So I waved my hand a little and signed "A. S. L." a couple of times until somebody noticed. She said, "Sign language? OK, we'll try." I wasn't entirely with it, so I'm sure that my ASL wasn't the greatest, but I managed to get across that I wanted the tubes taken out of my throat. They said they couldn't do that yet. That wasn't the answer I was looking for so I struggled some more. There were a lot of other nastier things I was attempting to sign that they didn't understand. Most of the four letter descriptions I had for my situation either didn't come across or were ignored. Obviously, the anesthesia and I weren't getting along very well, but I really doubt that anybody does very well after fourteen hours. Besides, how many other surgeries are that long? Then I felt something around each of my legs. *Now I'm bound hand and foot? Seriously? Where is the guy who promised me that I wouldn't be bound?* I really struggled at that point. As we saw from my wife's journal earlier, those were the circulation sleeves around my legs, not restraints. I guess at that point my whacked-out brain was ready to believe just about anything, so they were restraints as far as I was concerned and I wanted them off. Now.

You may notice that Kay didn't even mention the sign language in her journal, even though she counted exactly how many pieces of Jello I puked on the nurse, but I have confirmed with her that it happened. It just evidently wasn't a terribly important event given what was happening. I remember it vividly, even though it obviously didn't last very long.

They finally got me calmed down again. I waved my hand some more and pantomimed writing this time. They got me a pen and paper and I began to write. I let my feelings be known in no uncertain terms. Tie me up, will you? You'd be amazed at the great four letter vocabulary you can come up with even in the state that I was in. Finally, I wrote, "I didn't sign up to be restrained- no way, no how." Keep in mind that I still couldn't see, I was really pissed, I was tied to my bed, and I was writing on a piece of paper someone was holding under my hand for me. I am still proud of my ability to write in those circumstances. I'm not so proud of some of the content of the writing, but just exactly what did you expect from someone as frightened as I was? Besides, not only can I sail a boat from point to point, I can do it while spouting a foul fountain of outbursts that would make a one-eyed pirate blush. So I guess the nasty language was no big surprise.

You can tell from my description of these first few minutes of being awake that I was frightened and felt very alone. The person trying to interpret my ASL rantings and holding the paper (and folding it over and over again to try to hide from the nurses all the nasty things I was saying about them) was my wife. I didn't discover this for weeks. She assumed that I recognized her voice and just figured I knew it was her. I'm sorry to say that I didn't. But I can tell you that it would have been a huge comfort to me to know she was there. I'm guessing I would have been much easier to deal with if I had known. She has a way of talking to me that can get me calmed down quickly. I guess she's the Chris Whisperer or something. Imagine how much easier that would have made things for the hospital staff. I'm sure thrashing patients aren't a lot of fun for them, either. So for any of you headed for surgery, make sure your loved ones identify themselves and get a positive response from you that you understand who they are. It's completely possible that she told me it was her and I just didn't comprehend, being in the stupor I was. In my case, it just goes down as another fun story to tell. There are a lot of eyes that roll when I break that story out, "...so there I was strapped to the bed..."

We got through all the fussing and fighting and the nurse asked me to breathe by myself through the stupid tube to prove I was ready to have it taken out. "Breath as hard as you can out the tube, Mr. Miller," she said to me. I basically just blew bubbles with it. That was apparently enough since, thankfully, they took it out. If you had told me that I woke up at 8:00am and asked me what time they took out my breathing tube? I would have told you it was before 9:00am. But as we saw in Kay's journal notes, it wasn't until almost noon. Even now, years later, I still would swear up and down that it couldn't have been more than an hour.

Kay finally explained to me why I couldn't see. The bandages were covering my eyes. I finally got calmed down enough that they took the restraints off my wrists. Or maybe they just didn't need the restraints once the tube was out. Things were getting better now that I was untied, the tube was out of my throat, and I could at least see a little bit. My vision was still blurry, but I could deal with that for now.

The rest of my stay in the Neuro ICU was not a whole lot of fun. I was on all sorts of pain medications, I was still working off the effects of the anesthesia, and I felt like I had been through the deepest level of hell from the struggle when I woke up. I still did my best to get it together. A nurse came in (Nurse Kristina) to give me my pills for some other medications I was supposed to take orally. I'm not a spectacular pill taker at the best of times, and I explained that to her. She kindly asked me to try since I needed to take my medication. I tried, but I immediately vomited all down the front of both of us. When had I had any chicken broth? I didn't remember having that much chicken broth, but it came up anyway. I was really embarrassed about puking on the nurse. Barfing on women has never been the best way to begin any type of relationship, even the one between nurse and patient. They usually prefer intelligent conversation while you look in their eyes, or holding the door open for them or something. I didn't figure vomiting all over her was going to win me any brownie points, but I was so tired afterward that I just crashed for a while.

I got some rest for a while and was examined by my doctors and their residents and students. It seemed like things were getting better. Maybe this wouldn't be so bad. Then the nurse came in with more pills. I puked all over her again. I was completely mortified. At this point I don't think I was her favorite patient. The next time, they gave me some anti-nausea medication in my IV before I tried to eat or take pills. It was like magic. I became a huge fan of Zofran from then on.

This was about the point where the reality of what my recovery was going to be like started to set in. I have mentioned the term "temporary facial paralysis" a couple of times before. The doctors had told me this was to be expected after the surgery. They were right. When they had first told me that it would be like that, I wasn't too worried. Temporary facial paralysis doesn't sound too bad, right? Again, let's talk about reality. The left side of my face didn't move. It felt like it was moving, but it didn't move at all. Tear production in my left eye had stopped because of the paralysis, so they had to put an ointment in my eye to keep it from drying out and then tape it closed. I could only imagine what other joys awaited me as we moved forward.

Night time in the neuro-ICU wasn't a whole lot of fun, either. The night nurse was charged with checking my blood sugar levels and she came in several times during the night and pricked my fingers for the sample. Big deal, you think. Millions of people have to do that every day! But those millions of people weren't on heavy duty narcotics. I could not for the life of me figure out why having someone take my pulse would hurt my fingers so much. *Mmmm, don't want to wake up... Sure you can take my hand- Ouch! What the hell?* On one of her last trips in to check on me, I finally was coherent enough to ask her what she was doing and she explained. Oh. Well that makes more sense. Then I fell asleep again. The sounds coming from the rest of the neuro-ICU weren't good. I was lucky enough to be one of the better cases in the unit, but that didn't make the sounds any easier to listen to. The other patients around me were victims of strokes, cerebral hemorrhage, and other brain injuries. I really felt bad for some of the people in there and their families. Not sounds I'll ever forget.

During my second night in the ICU, another night nurse came in with some warm washcloths to help me get cleaned up a little. I was then moved from the Neuro ICU to a regular hospital bed in the Neurology ward.

Part 3 - Recovery

9 – IN THE HOSPITAL

My room in the Neurology ward was nice. I was really glad to have a single room, since I don't always get along really well with people during the best of times, let alone during my recovery from brain surgery. The nurses even brought in a cot for my wife to be able to stay with me. Everyone was very accommodating. The nurses had adjusted my bandages for me so that my eyes were almost completely uncovered. There was still something wrong with my vision that made it all blurry and I was still pretty out of it, but it made a big difference. So I could at least see that the room was private, well lit, there was a television (that I couldn't focus my eyes on), and the Neurology ward nursing staff seemed great. I remember hoping that I wouldn't vomit on any of them. I'm sure that the whole episode of me puking on poor Nurse Kristina had become a story that made its way to the Neurology ward. How embarrassing. The doctors and residents continued to stop in to see me on a regular basis.

Since I was now in a regular hospital room, I was also able to have visitors. My older sister, Pat, and her boyfriend, Bob, stopped by to visit several times. It was really nice to have them there. At one point Bob wondered why it was so important that they be there if all I did was sleep. I can assure you that it's important for people to keep in mind how nerve wracking it can be to be loopy from all the drugs and wake up to find yourself alone in a strange place. It really is nice to wake up to see a familiar face once in a while. I woke up several times during their visits over those first couple of days and can't begin to tell you how comforting it was to have someone there. I would open my eyes and wonder where I was, then glance over and see that Pat and Bob were there and make some vague effort at communication before nodding off to sleep again. The key was that I realized that I wasn't alone.

Pat and Bob visiting also allowed Kay some extra flexibility to go home and get some sleep, take care of personal and household needs like bills, shower, get a change of clothes, and just get a break from the stress of being at the hospital. I think sometimes she just needed a chance to catch her breath. I've explained how stressful the build-up to having the surgery was for both Kay and me. Now that the surgery was over, all I had to concentrate on was getting better. That was all I could concentrate on, given my condition. My wife's stress levels didn't go down at all, though. She was dealing with trying to be near me at the hospital as much as she could to provide support to me, trying to keep family and friends updated, keep all the stuff at home taken care of, and still not forget about the job she would have to go back to after her leave was up. There are a lot of men who grumble about their wives for trivial things, but my situation made me glad to have such an amazing woman by my side.

Dr. Kim, his residents, and his students came in one of the early days to see how I was doing. They wanted to change my bandage and also get a look at the incision site. Kay was there and was able to watch from behind the doctors. She had been extremely good at taking all of the medical stuff in stride and didn't stop here. The only thing that changed on her face was that her eyes got noticeably wider when she got a look under the bandage. That was the only outward sign when she saw the surgical site. Unfortunately, I know my wife pretty well and could read a lot into the wide eyes. She doesn't exactly have the greatest poker face of all the players at the table. Her face almost always shows exactly what she's feeling or thinking. *Uh-oh. If she thinks it looks that bad, it must be pretty scary. But all the doctors seem to like what it looks like. That must mean that while they look good, there are a LOT of stitches.* There were definitely a lot of stitches if the sight of it was enough to make her eyes widen like that. But we knew it was going to be a pretty serious incision. Remember that just the initial description of it had caused me to swoon like a Victorian lady.

Even there in my nice, private hospital room, the night time brought its own set of trials. There was a bulletin board under the television in my room with some posters pinned to it. They were mostly posters about the importance of washing your hands and that kind of thing. I guess it was just typical hospital public service reminder subject matter. I woke up in the middle of that first night to find that a picture of a person on one of the posters had turned into a nasty feline-looking monster. No lie. Even with the excuse of all the painkillers this one is just bizarre. It was obviously a trick of the shadows and light, but the woman pictured on one of the posters had turned into a monster that vaguely resembled a panther. And her hand that she was holding up to remind you to wash well and often? It was now a big paw with long scary talons on it. The monster was a mix of a lot of purple, yellow, and gray colors. *Don't look at the monster. The monster isn't real. Just don't look at the monster. Just look away and calm down, then go back to sleep.* I had to turn my head to the side and stare at the wall or I was going to have a panic attack. What a great headline that would be: "Man dies of heart attack in hospital after complaining of scary monster on poster." Staring at the wall seemed like the best way for me to calm down. Eventually I did, and I was able to get back to sleep.

I asked Kay right away the next morning to cover that poster up or flip it over or something. I explained why when she asked. I got a blank stare in response. I can laugh about it now since I can only imagine how ridiculous it must have sounded to have a grown man asking his wife to cover up the picture of the woman that became a scary monster at night. I'm sure she was thinking she was going to have to start checking under the bed for me when I went to sleep. You never know, there could be another bad monster hiding under there, too! I appreciate the fact that she didn't say anything or laugh at me; she just covered up the poster. My sister brought in a picture of her dog, Pippy, to hang on the bulletin board. He's my little buddy, but he actually is a monster. It's a wonder he didn't turn into a good elf or something at night. Having a picture of that silly dog hanging in my room was a big comfort.

I still think the monster story is kind of fun, even though it scared the wits out of me at the time. I was less amused with the paper towel dispenser. The scary poster said to wash your hands, right? So every doctor, resident, student, nurse, or guest would wash their hands as soon as they came in the room. The paper towel dispenser was one of the models that senses your hand in front of it, a motor whirs, and a paper towel pops out. Over. And over. And over again. I heard that machine whirring and ejecting paper towels at all hours. Now when I am out somewhere and have just finished washing my hands and reach up for a towel I can't help but give a little shiver at the sound that machine makes when I wave my hand in front of it. I get my towel and move on as quickly as possible. The temptation to smash the thing into little tiny pieces has come up once or twice. How ridiculous is it that I have an emotional reaction to a paper towel dispenser? I am very thankful that they have not become fashionable to have in private homes. I wish they would go out of style in public places.

And speaking of pictures, I almost forgot the coolest picture over on the table across from my hospital bed. I had a picture of Chaka Khan with the handwritten message, "Get Better Chris- Love + God Bless, Chaka Khan" on it. How cool is that? And how on earth did it end up on the table in my hospital room next to all the other well wishes? My sister had been on the train from New York to DC the weekend before and had seen a woman traveling with what seemed to be a small entourage or body guards. Out of curiosity, Pat looked a little closer and saw that it was Chaka Khan. She went over to Ms. Khan and introduced herself and told her about my situation and upcoming surgery. Chaka Khan very graciously took out a publicity photo card and a Sharpie and wrote me that kind message. I thought it was pretty cool.

By now I was making small dents in regular hospital meals. The food was great. I found myself checking the clock as mealtimes approached with anticipation of something tasty. Anybody who equates hospital food with something bad has not stayed at Georgetown University Hospital. The meals and meal service staff were both top notch. But I was interrupted one morning by a couple of people from the Physical Therapy department. Sure! I'd love to get out of this bed. They were very helpful and asked how I was feeling and very gingerly and gently got me up out of bed and seated in a chair that they had pulled over. We talked some more about how I was feeling, then they left. *Hey wait, where are you going? You can't leave me here! I'm recovering from surgery, can't you tell?* I guess they missed the part where I was still in the chair. I learned much later from a student while I was in Physical Therapy for my face that this was a very common practice. The idea is that you have to get back into bed on your own. I have theorized that the thought is along the lines of leaving you stranded there in the chair, you'll find some amazing strength of will and stand up and shout out-loud that you've been saved, that you're cured. Not really. I learned from the PT student that they are just trying to help you feel more independent. To help you realize that you aren't as helpless as you feel. Personally? I think it's kind of a crappy thing to do. I wasn't in very good shape yet. My eyes still wouldn't focus quite right, which made it hard to get a feel for depth perception. Not to mention the fact that the tumor and the surgery both involved my vestibular nerve, which is a critical balance component. I would have preferred they stay and help get me safely back into bed. Wishes and nickels and all that, I suppose. Kay and I struggled and got me back into bed. She helped me to get back over to the bed and get me lined up to ease back down into bed. I kind of missed on the whole "ease" thing and ended up more falling back into bed. Luckily, I didn't hurt myself. I did start getting out of bed once in a while after their visit, and that helped make me feel better. The whole incident still left me with a bad taste in my mouth. I just thought it could have been handled better for a patient with balance and eyesight problems.

Being in the hospital was really depressing sometimes, and I felt like I needed something to focus on after I got out of the hospital and got through the rest of my recovery. I came up with doing a one-hundred mile "Century" bicycle ride. What better way to prove to myself that I had fully recovered than riding one-hundred miles on a Saturday? You can just ignore the part where I had never ridden more than about twenty-five miles before. Having a goal to think about and focus on was a huge help. There were some days where thinking about getting out of the hospital and riding my bike really got me through the day.

I would suggest having a good goal to anyone dealing with a difficult hospital stay and continuing recovery. Or any physical or emotional struggle for that matter. It will give you something positive to look forward to! If your goal includes some physical activity, even better. That part of it will make the fact that you are stuck in bed a little easier to deal with because you can imagine yourself out working towards achieving your goal. It doesn't have to be epic. Maybe it can be going for a walk on a favorite route, or playing softball at the community picnic, or running a 5k. Heck, your goal might be to do an Ironman event- just be sure that you set a realistic timetable for achieving whatever goal you set for yourself. As my story continues, you'll see that I wasn't going to be doing any Ironman events or Century bike rides anytime soon. These needed to be long term goals.

Some of the things that happened to me in the hospital just weren't as funny to me as they were to other people. Remember the discussion about walking in to find your patient hooked to all sorts of tubes and wires and hoses? And there had been a bit of an embarrassing little incident? As I was progressing through my hospital stay, it occurred to me that I hadn't urinated that I could remember since we came in on Tuesday for the surgery. I had basically been in bed since then. Was I just not remembering getting up to use the bathroom? That didn't seem right. I hadn't been that out of it for at least a day or two. They had given me a big 32oz mug with a straw for water. I was going through several refills per day. There was no way I could hold it that long, could I? I asked Kay about it. I got that same blank stare that I had gotten when I asked about covering up the poster with the monster on it. Uh-oh. "Are you serious?" Yes, otherwise I wouldn't have asked. "Sweetie, look under the blanket. Do you see that tube going under your gown?" Yeah, but what does that tube sticking out of my gown that goes down over my leg have to do with... Oh. I get it. Lovely. Thankfully I was still drugged up enough to not notice her working really hard at keeping a straight face and not burst out laughing. It did explain a lot.

That story about the Foley catheter and my wife's reaction to my questions about it might have been kind of funny. I'm fine with us all having a good chuckle at my lack of understanding. Ha-ha. It got far less funny a couple of days later. A young nurse came into my room with a purpose and informed me that it was time to remove the Foley catheter. I think it's pretty obvious from my previous naive questions to my wife that I had never had one of these before, nor was I awake when it was inserted. So I was a little vague on the details with regard to the process of removal. I politely asked if it was going to hurt. The nurse said that she didn't know because she had never had one before. In my research for writing my story, I made the mistake of doing a Wikipedia search on the Foley catheter.

Oops. Those pictures have scarred me for life, but I now know that it's a "man only" bit of medical accessory. I guess that little omission on the nurse's part got past me, and so once I got the tears wiped off of my cheeks and my dignity realigned, I suggested she tell the next person who asked that it did indeed hurt. It hurt a lot! Without being too graphic, she just pulled it out as gently as she could. I honestly can say that I can think of nothing more emasculating than having an attractive young nurse reach up under your gown with both hands, get a good grip on both you and the tube, and pull out your catheter. Anyway.

Getting the catheter out was a step towards getting me more mobile. They brought me a walker to help me get around. The walker was a great tool for me while my balance was getting itself sorted back out. Add in some assistance from Kay, Pat, Bob along with smiles and waves from the nurses at their station, and I was able to stumble and dodder all the way around the ward. It was like track and field in super slow motion. The nurse's station made a kind of infield with a wide aisle all the way around it. I would leave my room taking two little steps at a time, then a move forward with my walker, then two more little steps and another move with the walker. Walking a total of about one-hundred fifty feet took me almost ten minutes and left me feeling exhausted for hours. I wasn't going to complain, though, since I was up and moving and not lying in the hospital bed for at least short periods of time.

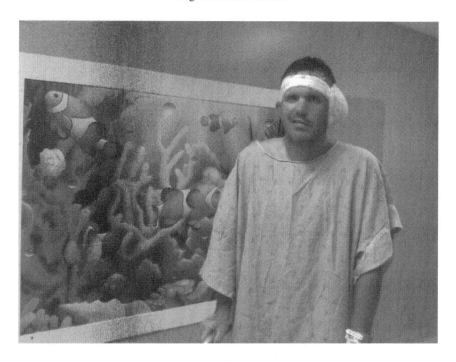

I also had to get up and use the en-suite bathroom now, giving me an opportunity to see myself in the mirror for the first time. I looked terrible. The bandage they had on me wrapped around my head a couple of times and it held a bundle of gauze in place to try to keep a constant pressure on the incision site. It looked like half of Princess Leia's hairdo. When you mixed that with several days of scruffy beard growth, my hospital gown, my tan grippy socks, and my walker- it left me looking a little less than GQ. I was also able to sneak a peek under the bandage at the surgical site. Why do I keep doing things like this? Note to self: hey self? looking under the bandage at this point is not a smart thing.

My time in front of the mirror also gave me my first look at what the reality of "temporary paralysis" meant. Along the way to this point, I had gotten the impression that things with my face weren't very good. I struggled to eat. Food had been consistently falling out of my mouth. I could only use the right corner of my mouth to drink out of a straw. It just wasn't possible to get my lips to work correctly and get a good seal around the straw if I tried it anywhere other than the right corner. I knew something wasn't quite right. I even was aware of the concept of looking like a stroke victim. They had warned me about the fact that there would be some drooping and flaccidity in my face before the surgery. But it didn't prepare me for what I saw in the mirror.

The terminology of "temporary paralysis" doesn't sound that bad when you hear it. It seems like you just won't be able to move that side as well. That part is true, but it doesn't end there. It also means that your facial muscles on that side aren't getting the instructions to hold things in place. So everything sags. Still not a big deal? The good side doesn't have that problem. And there's nothing you can do to either side to compensate at all. I'll come back to this subject again, but it continued to become very clear to me that things weren't going to be as simple as they seemed.

Being able to get up and go to the bathroom also meant that I could brush my teeth! It had been four or five days at this point since I had brushed my teeth. I had been under for the first twenty-four hours, I'd been sleeping far more than normal, and I had vomited several times in the past couple of days. I had the worst case of morning breath imaginable. My teeth were downright furry. I quickly discovered that brushing wasn't an activity that glossed over my facial paralysis, either. Not being able to control the left side of my mouth meant that I made a horrible mess the first time I tried to brush my teeth. There was foamy toothpaste mess oozing all over my chin and down the front of my gown before I even realized what was happening. I quickly figured out that I needed to hold my mouth directly over and facing the sink. That way everything just drooled right on out to the sink, thus eliminating the middle man of my chin and gown. Rinsing was even worse. The concept of swishing water around in your mouth has a basic prerequisite of being able to keep your lips sealed. I did not come to the activity armed with that ability. I swished around the right side a little, then pushed the water back over to the left side of my mouth expecting that it would stay put and just rinse off my teeth. That wasn't exactly the actual result. I sprayed toothpaste and water all over. They certainly hadn't mentioned this in the temporary paralysis brochure.

I concentrated on becoming more mobile over the weekend and could feel myself starting to get a little stronger. My lap times around the ward got faster and I even managed a couple of two lap sessions. On Monday morning, the doctors suggested that I could probably go home later that day. I was pretty excited to go home after spending a week in the hospital. I missed my dog, and the comfort of just being in my own space. I would not be sad to be leaving all the poking and prodding behind. I had been extremely well cared for during my stay at Georgetown by all the doctors, nurses, and staff, but I was still looking forward to getting home.

The anticipation was running pretty high immediately after they told me that discharge that day was a possibility, and continued to grow with every passing minute. I was going to be able to sleep in my own bed. I was going to be left alone for the most part since there wouldn't be a nursing staff there to be poking and testing and monitoring. I had gone from spending most of my days alone with the dog during the daytime to being surrounded with people constantly. It was a great feeling to know that I was being looked after so well, but it was also a lot of stress to be constantly in the spotlight.

There was some worry on Monday about something dealing with my endocrine system. A level of some sort that wasn't quite right required urine samples and a lot of testing. The doctors were going to consult with another specialist in the hospital to be sure everything was going to be OK when I went home. This made the normal discharge process a little more complicated. We discovered the need to be your own advocate during the discharge process. The nice people at Georgetown would have been more than happy to have me stay for another day or so to be sure that everything was perfect. But for me, once they suggested that going home was a real possibility, I was all about it. It just took a little bit of a balance of persistence and patience. I asked every staff member who came into my room that day how the discharge process was coming along. Every nurse, every doctor, every anybody who walked in my room. At one point we resorted to asking people walking past my room. I made sure to be polite about it. When I felt like my patience might not last, Kay would ask instead. She wanted to be gone from the hospital almost as much as I did. I'm sure it was probably a little annoying to the nurses and staff, but it helped make the day go faster for us.

We learned another important lesson that day. Make sure you get any prescriptions filled at the hospital pharmacy long before they might close. The double-checking of issues with my endocrine system along with the normal process of patient discharge took most of the day. I didn't get wheeled out of the hospital until just after 6:00pm. The hospital pharmacy hours were only until 6:30pm. We had planned on just picking up the prescriptions on the way out of the hospital campus, but by the time we got me loaded into the car and got to the pharmacy it had closed. I now didn't have any pain medication to go home with. It was not a situation that either Kay or I were prepared to deal with. All of my energy was being spent just trying to stay upright. And we knew that I wouldn't do well without pain medication when we got home and the current dose I was on wore off.

This had my wife a little flustered for the ninety minute drive home in the middle of Washington rush hour traffic. She was on the phone with Dr. Kim trying to make arrangements for another prescription to be called in to our local pharmacy near home. Her worry over me being in pain along with the regular frustrations of traffic added up to a pretty aggressive car ride on the way out of town. The time in the car was also the longest I had been upright in the past week and I was still terribly woozy. Using the Mario Andretti method of navigating the narrow and crowded Georgetown streets and then the beltway around DC wasn't very comfortable for me. The jerky ride of the car started to give me a nasty headache and I had to ask Kay to please calm down for my sake. I understood her frustration and would have been driving much the same way if the situation were reversed, but I really needed a smooth ride home to keep the pain and dizziness in check. She took a nice, deep breath and the rest of the ride home was much smoother. We were both relieved to be going home.

10 – BACK HOME

We made it home in one piece, but I was a complete mess. I was exhausted and starting to get grumpy because I was getting hungry. Even the much calmer ride home had still taken a huge amount of energy out of me. It also gave me a nasty headache just from the little bit of movement that the ride made for my head. I asked Kay to fix me something to eat. My wife is a great person and a very successful business executive, but let's just say that she's not a spectacular cook. I usually do all the cooking at home, but obviously that wasn't going to happen for a while due to my physical condition. She was kind enough to make me some tomato soup. In my haste to have something to curb my growing hunger, I unwisely suggested that she make it in the microwave oven rather than her preferred stove-top method. Important tip: shut your mouth when someone is trying to fix you something to eat. We ended up with soup exploding all over the microwave and me sitting quietly at the kitchen island eating luke warm, clumpy, tomato soup trying desperately to avoid making my wife any more angry than I already had. The soup was still good enough to make me feel a little bit better afterward.

We had been smart enough to ask the surgical team what sort of preparations we could set up at home to make things easier during my recovery. They had said that I would not be able to negotiate stairs for the first week or two that I was at home and would probably need the walker to get around for at least the first few days.

Am I ever glad we asked! We had rearranged some furniture and moved a bed downstairs into our living room before going to the hospital the week before. It was great. I could get to the bathroom, the kitchen, and back to bed pretty easily with the help of my walker.

There are some other things that we could have done to make things easier for those first few days. We've seen what happened when the normal cooking routine was interrupted: a section of the kitchen ended up coated from the ten megaton tomato soup bomb. It would have been helpful to have had some simple, easy-to-fix foods stocked in the house. A frozen casserole or two would have been super. We ended up moving a table in next to the bed to hold things like a glass of water, pictures, a book, and "Get Well Soon" cards. My treasured get well message from Chaka Khan was prominently placed among the cards from family and friends we actually knew. My wife didn't understand my fascination with the whole Chaka Khan thing, but then she didn't have a get well message from a ten-time Grammy Award winner, did she? The thirty-two ounce mug that they sent me home from the hospital with was a great thing to have. It had a sealed lid and a straw. Having only half of your mouth work makes an adult model sippy-cup a real asset around the house. I liked that it made me slightly more independent those first few days. I could just sit up a little bit and reach over to the side table and get a drink of water. I was really thirsty during the first week home. I think it might have been from the medications.

Speaking of the medications, I discovered another joy of the heavy duty pain medications and anesthesia when I went to use the bathroom that first night back home. To put it delicately, the anesthesia and pain medications had a net effect of giving me a serious case of constipation. I hadn't had a bowel movement since before I went in the hospital and even though I hadn't eaten a whole lot during my stay; it had still been a week! I know you've just made a comment about how this is really more than you wanted to know. Agreed. But any modesty I had before all of this was gone. Long gone. Any tiny little bit of innocence I might have still clung to was painfully removed with the Foley catheter. Besides, you're about to see that the constipation actually plays a very important role in my story.

Given the huge amount of narcotic pain killers that my body had processed over that week, my first trip to the bathroom on Monday evening, a little while after we got home from the hospital, was a bit of a struggle. Any exertion on my part had a really odd side effect. Every time I strained, I felt something wet dripping down the back of my neck and off my head onto the floor. I can assure you that it was not something that had ever happened to me before I went to the hospital. I reached back and touched the wetness and my fingers came away with a clear, viscous, odd smelling fluid on them. I rubbed it between my fingers and tried to figure out what it was. Whatever it was, it would drip slowly down the back of my neck when I was relaxed, but when I strained at all it would run in rivulets from under my bandage. This continued any time I struggled for the duration of my stay in the bathroom. When I came out, I asked my wife about it. My bandages were soaked with the fluid, the rug in front of the toilet had a large spot of it, and my shirt and pants had several damp patches on them. There had been a fair amount of it leaking from wherever it had come from. It wasn't blood, so it didn't seem very serious. It was a mystery neither one of us had the energy to deal with. We should have called the hospital and asked. All of those things I mentioned above, from my bandages to the bathroom rug, were soaked with CerebroSpinal Fluid. You might have heard of it referred to before as brain fluid. We were completely clueless as to what it might be at the time. It had been a long and stressful day getting out of the hospital, home, fed, and all we wanted to do was get some rest. So I went to bed with a wet, slimy, and now cold bandage on. We could worry about that part of it later, it was time to get some sleep.

I look back on the concept and shake my head at having what probably totaled somewhere around four fluid ounces of brain fluid leak from my skull while I was straining on the toilet. I cannot believe sometimes how stupid and naive we were about the realities of medical things. Absolutely nothing should have been leaking from my surgical site, but we just completely ignored something really bizarre leaking from it. We really were tired of doctors and hospitals and everything at that point, but how stupid could we be? We'll see shortly just how stupid we were to ignore this incident, but in the meantime we had plenty more adventures in front of us.

Getting into bed that first night home, the painkillers gave me some bizarre dreams. You thought the woman on the poster turning into a monster was strange? That first night, sleeping in the bed in the middle of our living room, I dreamed that I was unrolling a spool of wire out of a cylindrical container of ice cream. Sounds like a real winner, you say? You'd be absolutely right. The wire was the big, thick, black stuff they use in high-voltage electricity transmission lines. The container of ice cream was about the size of a five gallon bucket, and had the wire neatly coiled inside. The ice cream made the wire cold to the touch and slimy. I vividly remember the grimace I made, grossed out in my dream by how sticky and wet my hands were getting. One turn of wire out of the bucket- don't ask me what I was doing with it after I took it out of the bucket, I have no idea- then another turn out of the bucket, and another. I was about four or five turns into the process when I jolted awake. Something on my head felt peculiar. I reached up with my left hand to check on my bandage and found it missing. I touched stitches instead.

It turned out that I had really been unwrapping my cold, slimy bandage off of my head in my sleep. Uh-oh. That isn't good. I woke my wife and told her what had happened. She very patiently got out our bandaging materials and got my head wrapped back up. She did a heck of a good job of it even though it was the middle of the night. She managed to get me looking an awful lot like Princess Leia again. We were fortunate that Kay was better the first time around at bandaging than she was at making canned soup in the microwave oven. I'm sure she was nervous about having to bandage me back up. I can only imagine the things going through her mind while she was getting my head tightly wrapped again. Luckily, I was able to sleep without any more bandage-removing dreams for the rest of the night. I think that is by far the strangest dream I have ever had, before or since. Let's hope I keep it that way.

The next morning I found my pillow completely soaked with the strange, slimy goo that had been leaking out from under my bandage the night before. At first I thought I had just drooled all over it, since it had such a similar feel against my cheek. I remembered the fluid leaking incident from the night before and had an "ewwwwww" moment. We still didn't know what the stuff was, but I wasn't thrilled about having my face shoved in it any longer than necessary. I was still struggling with being upright for too long or doing too much moving around, so I asked Kay to wash my pillow in the washing machine for me. I figured a clean pillow might give me a fresh start towards an uneventful night's sleep, given the unusual experiences of the night before. There might have been a part of me that just didn't want to sleep on the crusty pillow that I was sure I was going to have once all that goop dried.

Washing my pillow thrust my wife back into the domestic arena that she struggles with sometimes. I waited for her to ask my opinion this time rather than give it unsolicited like I did with the soup. Fool me once, as the saying goes. When she came in and asked, I suggested that she just put the pillow in by itself in our front load machine and wash it on a normal warm cycle with a little laundry detergent. Nothing complicated. In fact, the machine actually has a cycle called "Normal," which was what I wanted her to use. We were in the kitchen a little while later, trying to get me some time out of bed, when I smelled the odor of something burning coming from around the corner in the laundry room. I hobbled in there to see what was happening and saw through the window in the washing machine door that the drum was moving around while the pillow wasn't. I hit the pause button on the machine, opened the door, and was presented with a strong odor of smoke. I pulled the pillow out to find that my wife had closed the corner of the pillow in the washing machine door when she closed it. The drum spins at some pretty high speeds and produced so much friction that it was working desperately to light my pillow on fire. It was actually charred on the corner that had been closed in the door. I would bet that people light their laundry on fire in the dryer all the time, but I'm guessing that my wife is one of the rare few that can almost start a fire in the washing machine with it full of water. We had a good laugh over it. We both know all too well what each of us brings to our relationship, and obviously the laundry skills don't fall into her column.

We had another stroke of luck in having friends who are professionals in the medical field. One of our nurse friends came over and changed the bandage the next day and showed Kay some tips for getting me bandaged up in case I had any more dreams about ice cream. A couple of days later, another nurse friend and her pharmacist husband stopped by to help with another bandage change and check on my progress. Having these medical professionals just double checking on me and helping with the bandages was really great. We felt pretty confident about how things were going with their help. Unfortunately, as much as their help was really appreciated, it turned out not to be a good situation later on. The dressing that had been put on my at the hospital was wrapped very specifically to keep a firm, constant pressure on the surgical site. We didn't realize this and did not convey that to our friends who were helping us. They didn't get the opportunity to see the original bandage application thanks to my rather industrious dreaming habits, so none of them could see how Dr. Kim had wanted the dressing to apply pressure to the surgical site. The bandages with less pressure ended up not being a good thing, as we will see in a few moments. I thank those two ladies very much for helping me and Kay and I will always be grateful for their willingness to provide their expertise. This particular bandaging job required a key piece of information that we did not provide them. Lesson learned: get instruction on the specifics (in writing, if possible) on any bandaging or wound care techniques.

My wife was kind enough to work from home for several days when I first returned home from the hospital. She had already been on leave for over a week during my hospitalization, and now she called in a couple of favors in order to telecommute for those first days back home so I could get to a point where I was a little more independent. There was one day that first week back that she really needed to go into the office for a particular meeting, so my sister volunteered to come out and visit me. Did I really need 'round the clock observation and company? Probably not. Was I glad that there was someone there in case I needed something? Heck, yes! Pat was even indulgent to the point of doing a little housework while she was there to try to make things a little easier for Kay now that we were back home. Or maybe I was just really boring company and vacuuming was better than watching me sleep.

I received quite a few cards wishing me a speedy recovery from all sorts of friends and family. One of them was even more unique than the Chaka Khan photo with her well wishes. A friend of my parents was an amazing artist and sent me a small watercolor painting of a schooner sailing vessel out on the water as a "get well" card from him and his wife. I was grateful for all of the cards and well wishes from everyone, but Herb's small painting was really touching. It was so typical of him and his wife to share his incredible talent in such an unassuming way. The generosity that it showed was typical of them, too. Herb had retired from painting a couple of years before and only worked on things he was personally interested in, which made this great card even more meaningful. Herb has since passed, leaving his special card as a cherished part of my small collection of his artwork.

We got a visit from our friends from Annapolis, Mark and Cindi, who had gone to Trader Joe's and brought us all sorts of yummy things to pack our refrigerator and freezer with. Most of the food was pretty simple heat-n-serve type meals which made things much easier on us for the next week or so in the kitchen. It was a really nice switch from Kay's tomato soup.

Bogey came home from his stay with the friends who had kindly been dog-sitting for us while I had been in the hospital. Being a greyhound, Bogey is seventy pounds of lanky sharp angles. Bogey is also seventy pounds of pure cuddly love. He is very cognizant of when you are not feeling well and does his best to provide top notch snuggle support. He did a great job of very gently snuggling with me and just being my partner during my first couple of weeks home. "Nurse Bogey" was great company during the day while my wife was working in her office down the hall.

We also got visits from more of our friends in those first couple of weeks back home. It was great to have people take the time to come see us. The baked goods, peanut butter cups, and vita-malt were a bonus. I have unhealthy obsessions with a couple of things in life: peanut butter and vita-malt. I think most people can understand the peanut butter fetish, but the vita-malt thing leaves most of my friends just scratching their heads. We enjoy spending time in the southern Caribbean islands on vacation every couple of years and I had gotten hooked on this particular drink on my first visit there. Vita-malt is a non-alcoholic malt beverage that I always compare to drinking liquefied Frosted Flakes cereal. Luckily, I had found it bottled by a Spanish foods specialty label and readily available in most grocery stores in the United States. I had smiled my one-sided smile about as big as it would go when some friends of ours came to visit and brought a basket filled with bottles of vita-malt and peanut butter cups. I was in heaven.

I had lost about fifteen pounds during my week in the hospital, but it didn't take me long to put it back on. It was fantastic to see everyone. And having everyone bring food or treats didn't hurt anything either! It was good for Kay to have some social interaction while I wasn't strong enough to get out of the house at all. I also was very appreciative of everyone being sympathetic to my situation, but not acting any different around me.

Our friends reacted really well to my situation. It was kind of them to take time out of their summer schedules and come out to visit us. They were also fantastic about taking my physical changes in stride. I looked like crap. My face was all droopy on the left side, I was blinking my eye manually with my left index finger, I didn't get around very well and tired easily, and I wasn't necessarily in the best of moods for all the visits, but nobody seemed to mind. I think they were all relieved that I was still around and looked like I would make my way back to some near semblance of the me they knew from a few weeks before.

It was a slow process, but I got a little stronger every day. Eventually I got to the point where I did not need the walker to get around. Instead, I staged it half-way between the living room, where the bed was still set up, and the kitchen. That way if I found myself in trouble while I was moving around, my walker was never far away. I managed to go up and down the stairs being careful to hold on tight to the railing. As soon as I could get up and down the stairs at will, we could stop sleeping in the living room. Both Kay and I were looking forward to any little thing that would indicate things were getting back to normal, even if it was just sleeping in the bedroom instead of the living room. It really seemed like this whole recovery process was going to be unpleasant, but we'd get through as best we could and just deal with it.

We went for my check-up visit with Dr. Kim, and he changed my bandage and scolded us a little because we had changed it. This was really kind of a difficult situation. Between being soaked with brain fluid and getting taken apart during my dream, the bandage I had left the hospital with had been ruined. It seemed to me that having some bandage was better than no bandage, but I understood Dr. Kim's concern that it wasn't the correct bandage that he wanted on me. He also decided to leave my stitches in for a while longer.

My continually increasing strength and endurance allowed us to venture out of the house a little bit. We went out for a bite to eat. We went to a couple of social events at the sailing club. None of our trips out were ever very long or were anything very strenuous, but we tried to get out enough to help reduce Kay's growing sense of cabin fever. Summer is usually a time when we spent a lot of time out sailing or doing other social activities. We hadn't been able to do any of that for weeks. So I would put on a decent looking bucket hat that would cover most of my Princess Leia bandage and try to ignore the stares of people out in public. That wasn't always an easy thing to do, so we often chose to find activities where we would be surrounded by friends that were just glad to see me recovering. Many of our sailing club friends that we hadn't seen in over a month were very happy to see us at the club picnic. Everyone was very understanding that I didn't have enough energy to be social for long, and took the opportunity to chat with Kay after stopping by to give me an affectionate pat on the shoulder or friendly kiss to let me know that I had been missed. Those simple gestures meant a lot to me. It was good to know that I was loved and cared for by my friends, and that they had been thinking about me while I had been working through the difficult physical part of my recovery.

I even decided to do some work that needed done at the rental house. I had a big pile of gravel delivered for the driveway and headed over there to shovel and rake it out. I didn't get very far. I quickly became exhausted and very dizzy, so I gave up and went home to rest. I called our friend, Rick, to see if he could give me a hand the next day around noon. I showed up at noon to find that Rick and his wife Cindy were just finishing up raking out the high spots of the new gravel driveway. They had shoveled and raked the entire pile out for me. What a relief! And what a nice thing to do. I really should not have been trying to do things like this. Instead, I should have been concentrating on making a slow and complete recovery. Thank goodness our friends realized this and were so willing to help!

Even with some efforts to get out of the house more, most of our free time was spent at home since I still didn't feel very good most of the time. I would get dizzy sometimes and I still tired quickly. I had tried getting out for a bike ride a couple of times, but I found that I just didn't have the strength. Poor Kay was going stir crazy. This was such a sudden and complete departure from our normal summer routine that it was a shock to her system. Besides, who wants to spend all their time with me when I was basically an invalid compared to what I had been just six weeks before. She had been so good and so patient with me that I decided I should just "suck it up" and go out for an upcoming casual sailing race weekend.

It had been about four weeks since my surgery when we took our boat out for a fun race with our sailing club. The course would take us about twenty miles up the Chesapeake Bay to the home port of another nearby sailing club. We would stay there for the night and return the next day. I knew that I would not have the strength to do most of the physical activities that I usually did on the boat, so we took along some of our friends as crew. Note this down as one of the smarter things we did. Kay is the captain on our boat, *Sequoia*. Just like at home, we each have a particular skill set that we specialize in on the boat. While she is excellent at the wheel, I work hard to make the sails work as efficiently as possible. Trimming the sails on the boat requires some intermittent, intense physical efforts, none of which I was going to be able to do on this particular day. We were glad to have Scott, Jenn, and Rob volunteer to join us so that I could just sit on the rail and not get overtired.

It was a sweltering day on the water and there was not much wind to sail, so we soon gave up the race and motored to our destination. I had started asking if we could give up and turn on the motor pretty early on, since being in the scorching heat with a tightly wrapped bandage on my head was no fun. The heat was causing me not to feel very well, either. Most of the other boats followed suit shortly after. I wasn't feeling fantastic, but I tried not to be a wet blanket. I knew that this was an important outing to help Kay get a little more social time in. We docked the boat when we arrived and all went to get cleaned up. I felt a little better after a nice cool shower, but I still wasn't feeling right. I went to the picnic that evening to socialize and I tried to put on a happy, albeit droopy, face.

One couple whom we often sail with was at the picnic, though they had been sailing up in New York and Rhode Island most of the summer and had missed my medical adventures. Dave is a retired physician who let me get about one minute into the back story about having the weird pressure and hearing loss on one side, when he said, "Did you have an Acoustic Neuroma or something?" How is that he needed one minute of description at a picnic while that witch-doctor of a nurse practitioner had multiple opportunities to figure it out and completely missed? Well, at least we knew that Dave's patients had always been in good hands.

I felt miserable the next morning when I woke up. It was hot again for the trip back, so the crew put up the awning on the boat and we just motored home. I was worthless; I just lay in the cockpit and tried not to be sick. The incredibly intense headache I had didn't make that easy given how hot and humid it was. Why did I feel so sick? Shouldn't I have been getting better?

I continued to descend into the deepest levels of being ill for the next week. I had follow-up appointments with my doctors scheduled for that Thursday which worked out great given how sick I felt. They would be able to help me. I was far too sick to drive myself anywhere, so yet another friend of ours offered to chauffeur me up to Georgetown on Thursday. I was glad that Joe was a smooth driver on Thursday since I was dizzy and ill. I felt faint when we arrived. We had to stop a couple of times on the short walk from the parking garage to the building entrance so that I could catch my breath and be sure of my balance. One time I had to stop in the middle of the small street running between buildings on the Georgetown medical campus. I just stood there in the crosswalk until I quit swooning. I felt bad for Joe being thrown into a situation where I was so ill, but I was certainly glad he was there in case I just dropped over in the middle of the street.

Both Dr. Kim and Dr. Jean were very concerned about my condition, but neither one could quite figure out why I felt so sick. They were worried about my surgical site, which had become swollen and puffy. I think they each considered having me admitted to the hospital right then. That probably would have been a smart thing to do, even though I would have been upset about it. They said that I should be back to almost normal levels of physical activity by this point, and yet obviously I was nowhere near normal. They suggested I give it a few more days and see if things turned around. I survived the trip home and thanked Joe for his help. I certainly wouldn't have been able to drive myself that day. He was just another friend showing how much he cared about me by taking time out of his busy schedule to help me in my time of need.

The next day, Friday, I felt dreadful. I was all but bed-ridden in the morning and felt nauseous. At about 9:00am, I made a stumbling dash for the bathroom and made it just in time to be violently ill a couple of times. Obviously something was wrong, so I called Kay. She had just gotten into the office, but she left right away to come back home. She must have heard in my voice just how sick I really was. I couldn't keep anything down. I tried some simple remedies like ginger ale to try to make my stomach feel better but they just came right back up. We made another call to my doctors and they suggested that I might want to come in to the emergency room if things did not improve. By late afternoon I had managed to keep down a couple of flavored ice treats like we had when we were kids on hot summer days. We decided that didn't necessarily count towards "getting better." It didn't take long to come to the conclusion that going up to Georgetown to the emergency room would be the smart thing to do.

Nothing in my story yet has happened without at least minor complications. This was no exception. We had offered to dog sit two greyhounds for our friends who had watched Bogey while I was in the hospital while they went out of town. Reciprocal dog watching is common with all dog owners, but it is especially common in the greyhound community. But what were we going to do with our Bogey and his guests, Bill & Betty? We called my sister, Pat, and she agreed to come stay with the three of them for the weekend at our house. Then we headed back into Georgetown on an early September Friday night to the emergency room.

11 – RETURN TO THE HOSPITAL

I felt truly horrible on the trip up to the Georgetown emergency room. I hadn't felt this crappy since I had gotten out of the hospital! Kay was doing her best to get us to the hospital quickly while still trying to make sure I didn't get sick. I was dizzy and nauseous, but managed to hold on until we got there. Almost there, anyway. We were about a half block from the turn onto campus and the ER when I told Kay to pull the car over. Now! I opened my door, leaned out, and retched up the freezer pops and ginger ale in the gutter. There was a small group of people walking in our direction down the sidewalk, and I can only imagine what a sad sight I looked to them. I'm sure I looked like some pathetic college student who couldn't hold his liquor on just the first weekend back to campus. I can honestly say that I was far too ill to worry much about what I looked like.

I was admitted to the ER pretty quickly. I think that having the Neurosurgery department call down to let them know that one of their patients is arriving must get you a high rank on the call list. We went through all the typical emergency room protocols: examination, testing, questions, pokes, prods and getting an IV inserted. I have mentioned my fear of needles a couple of times, and the IV insertion process in the ER did not do much towards changing my feelings about them. I had used the method where I just looked away and tried to ignore the fact that I was getting poked with a needle with a lot of success up to this point. I tried that again in this circumstance only to find that I was having to look away for a long time. I think maybe I was dehydrated from being so sick and my veins were hard to get to. There ended up being a little bit of pain and a fair amount of blood involved, but my IV was in.

The resident doctors from Neurosurgery came in and, of course, I knew the lead resident from my time spent in the hospital the month before. That was great, since I both liked him and had already developed a lot of trust in him. The trust in our doctor-patient relationship was going to be important for this visit. Even though I don't remember his name anymore, he was by far my favorite of the many resident doctors who worked with me. He was always very patient with my fears and frustrations and worked hard to communicate clearly with me to be sure that I understood what was going to happen to me. We talked through the issues and symptoms I was having while he examined me. From the initial tests and his observations, the team decided that they needed a CerebroSpinal Fluid (CSF) sample to test. Heck, a couple of weeks ago they could have just followed me into the bathroom, right? Or wrung out my bandage after I got it out of the ice cream container? In truth, I still didn't realize that CSF was the liquid that had been dripping down my neck that first night home.

Just how, exactly, does one go about getting a CSF sample? They said they'd really like me to have a spinal tap to get the sample. The only things I knew about spinal taps was that "this one goes to eleven" and that women giving birth had them and complained about how painful they could be. I had never given birth or had a drummer suddenly burst into flames, even though I had contemplated dousing a few in gasoline during my years spent playing in various rock bands, so I just kind of shrugged at them. They explained some of the complications that could occur, one of which was paralyzation- though it was quite rare. Oh fun. We didn't really see a lot of options here and we trusted the doctors, so we agreed to the spinal tap. I was feeling so miserable at this point that I would have done anything to feel better. They could have told me that they were going to pull out all my teeth with a pair of rusty pliers and I would have agreed just so long as it got rid of that damned headache.

Minutes after we got all the consent forms signed, the clock passed midnight. And it was now my birthday. Happy Birthday to me. Waiting for my spinal tap in the emergency room with a colossal headache hadn't exactly been on the short list of things I really wanted to do for my 36th birthday, but you play the hand you're dealt in life I guess. The head doctor on duty in the ER came in with another resident who was going to do the spinal tap. "Mr. Miller, this is resident doctor so-and-so who is going to do your spinal tap to get our CSF sample. It is? Really? Well Happy Birthday! Now if we can just get you to roll on your side and pull your pants down a little... just like that, perfect." At this point I really began to wonder what I had ever done to deserve this.

I was understandably nervous as they got out the needle and other equipment needed for the spinal tap. I was positive that this was going to make all the pain and discomfort up to this point seem like a walk in the park. Shoving that big, long needle into my back was surely going to be extremely painful. I was pleasantly surprised by the low level of pain. It wasn't fun, and I certainly wouldn't rush out to sign up for a spinal tap in my spare time or anything. But given the nervous anticipation that had been building in my mind, it ended up being pretty minor. I was just about to be exceedingly happy with the unanticipated lack of pain, when I discovered what feeling was going to be there in its stead. The spinal tap felt funky. It produced a warped feeling that ran through my body that wasn't painful, but it was very discomforting. That's really the only way I can describe it. We were a couple of minutes into the insertion of the needle when the doctor on duty said, "OK, Mr. Miller, you're going to feel an odd 'thump-thump' sensation." What the hell was she talking about? I mean, seriously, what could she possibly mean by... *thump-thump* Oh. Well. I guess she was talking about that. It was the strangest thing I had ever felt. I still have no idea what caused it, nor do I ever really want to know. All I can tell you is that it was freakishly odd. The feeling was a little like the stutter you get from dragging the toe of your sneaker as you walk, except that this was in my spinal column.

The resident with the needle got the sample drips of spinal fluid that he needed into a couple of vials to send off for testing and slowly eased out the needle. I checked to be sure I could still wiggle my toes. Yep, we got through it all without being paralyzed. They sent the samples off for lab work and tried to help me get comfortable while we waited. I got a little Zofran in my IV drip to settle my stomach. Don't ever say we don't learn our lessons well. Zofran had become a common part of my vocabulary at this point. I had even joined the Zofran fan page on Facebook. I thought it was funny that most of the other Zofran Facebook fans were nurses who didn't like being vomited on. I wondered if Nurse Kristina had joined the group. Probably.

The test results came back with a flurry of activity. A filter mask like you'd wear if you were working in a very dusty area was placed over my nose and mouth and Kay and I were rushed down the hall, past the inebriated freshman who was singing a happy little song on his gurney. He was the drunken student the people out on the sidewalk thought they had been snickering about. They moved Kay and I into a negative pressure room. The air pressure in a room like that is kept lower than that of the areas surrounding it so that there is no chance of any contaminants exiting the room, even when the door is open. Wait a minute. I've read about things like this in books, books like *The Andromeda Strain*, books about... epidemic. Oh crap. I was beginning treatment for the Bacterial Meningitis that my CSF samples tested positive for. It wasn't exactly the birthday I had anticipated. There hadn't been any gifts or cards waiting for me in my private little quarantine room when I arrived. Oh well, maybe later.

We stayed in the negative pressure room for a couple of hours until a room could be made ready upstairs in the main part of the hospital. I put my mask back on and they wheeled me up to my new room. The room was equipped with an air-lock. No lie. There was a small vestibule between my room and the hallway. It had a little less air pressure than the hallway, while having just a touch more pressure than my room. Understandably, I was being treated as a possible outbreak case of Meningitis. I was visited first thing by two hospital staff members wearing full bio-hazmat suits. Neither of them brought cake or a card. They were specialists in disease control and were trying to figure out if they had cause to worry about public safety. If I was just an isolated case I was obviously in danger from the Meningitis, but it didn't present a public threat. If I had contracted it from somewhere, there was a serious problem and they would need to get in touch with the Centers for Disease Control. I didn't realize that people in bulky yellow bio-suits, who were authorized to initiate a regional quarantine, could be so friendly. They were really very nice, while still clearly doing their job.

They took a look at the left side of my head and asked what the stitches were from. It was a little like being questioned by Darth Vader, though they didn't ask me any questions about a rebel base or any secret space station plans. I explained about the surgery and how I had gotten progressively more ill over the past couple of weeks. They left to go check my records and came back in a while later to ask a few more follow up questions about my surgery. I guess I had the answers they were looking for, since they took off their hoods and masks and apologized for the scare. They explained that the infection was obviously caused by my surgical site which meant that I did not pose any threat to the general populace. That made me feel better. I've been accused of being a menace to society by the occasional individual over the years, but being listed as a threat to the public hadn't really been on my birthday gift list. I could also check being questioned by someone in a full bio-hazmat suit off my bucket list. It wasn't nearly as much fun as you'd think.

That was how I began hospital stay number two.

12 – MENINGITIS TREATMENT

There I was back at Georgetown University Hospital being treated for Bacterial Meningitis with IV antibiotics. The antibiotics were working great, and I felt terrific within twenty-four hours. If I had known how quickly they could have made me feel better, I would have checked myself in the week before. I was put on a schedule of IV antibiotic treatment for one hour each morning and each evening. The only problem was the twelve hour gap in between the two treatments. I felt fine, but was still stuck in the hospital. We did get permission for me to leave my hospital room under the supervision of my wife for short periods. I felt like I was in Kindergarten since we had to ask the teacher (head nurse on duty) who in turn had to ask the principal (the Neurosurgery resident on duty) if I could go outside to play during recess. It was nice to be able to get out of the hospital room so that we could go for a short walk and have the occasional meal at the cafe across the parking lot from the hospital. I was still enjoying the food in the hospital, but it was a relief to get out of the room once in a while. We even snuck away from our approved outing area and stopped in the campus bookstore one day. I got a nice Georgetown Hoyas hat and a Georgetown Medicine t-shirt as souvenirs from my now multiple stays on campus. I thought about getting a set of hospital scrubs to wear as pajamas, but Kay and I agreed that a purchase like that might be pushing the limits of good Karma.

We got a visit from our friend, Rick, before he left town on business one day. He had a little extra time on his way to the airport and stopped in for a quick visit. I think our friends must have felt sorry for me having to be back in the hospital. They had all been so excited to have me back out socially in short doses and were evidently worried about me being admitted back into the hospital. It was nice to feel loved, especially given how terrible I had felt leading up to my re-admission to the hospital.

Aside from my antibiotic treatments, my daily schedule included having blood drawn a couple of times each day for testing. I had been slowly becoming desensitized a little bit to all the needles given the amount of poking and prodding I had gotten in the past month. I was really getting pretty good about having nurses stick me with them. My fears did cause a bit of trouble with my night nurse at one point, though. She came in and woke me up in the middle of the night to do a blood draw. No problem, I just turned my head the other way and looked at the wall. The nurse had a little trouble getting a vein in my arm and poked around a little bit more than I was used to. I woke up fully and started to pay a little more attention to what she was doing.

I don't know if my fear of needles is like other fears that people have, but I would guess it probably is. I get a little nervous and stare at the needle when a nurse or doctor holds it up. My heart-rate goes up and I start to breathe a little harder, but by that point usually whatever the needle was being used for is finished. No more needle. In cases like this when I'm presented with the needle for a longer time, I start to panic. My fear is obviously not rational; I'm not afraid of the pain the needle causes, since it doesn't cause much at all. Unfortunately, the panic that sets in soon turns to uncontrollable terror that manifests itself by me getting angry.

I had gotten to the panic stage when the nurse gave up poking around for a vein on my arm. I'm sure she was just having a tough night. We all have those, and normally I would have been more patient with her. I started to relax since I figured she'd just skip it and come back later to try again. Things all went terribly wrong when she said she was going to try to find a vein on the inside of my wrist. My unchecked terror found me jerking my hand away and telling her that there was no way in hell she was going to go digging around in my wrist with that needle! That was obviously not the best response for this situation, but I was scared. And I have a temper when I'm frightened or angry. Those two things added up to a heinous response from me since there was a needle involved. She kept trying to get me to give her back my wrist, which just made me more angry. I wasn't about to have her poking around in one of the most sensitive areas of the body with that needle for something as silly as a blood test that had been taken just a few hours earlier.

The nurse got flustered and left my room. She was replaced by the floor's head nurse on duty who asked what the problem was. I was trying to calm down and explained that I was terrified of needles and wasn't going to let my nurse poke me in the wrist with that needle. The head nurse was not exactly thrilled. I continued to expound on how frustrating it was to have the IV in my other arm that was only being used for two hours out of the day and yet I was still being stuck in the arm with needles to draw blood. Why couldn't they take the blood from my IV? She gave me several reasons why IV's were not normally used to extract blood, but agreed that we could try it, and thus we all worked to diffuse the situation. I noticed that I was assigned the head nurse every night for the duration of my stay. I had evidently been labeled as a difficult patient. The situation did make us wonder how much of a coincidence it was that the head nurse had a very commanding physical appearance. We were guessing it wasn't much of a coincidence at all. Her intimidating appearance certainly helped me to try to be as calm as possible, no matter how frightened and frustrated I was. Thankfully, there weren't any more altercations over blood draws. All efforts at blood sample extraction went off without a hitch for the rest of my stay.

Being in the hospital is no fun even when everyone is really nice and is taking great care of you. After a few days of being bored out of my mind, we called in the resident doctor on duty to talk about my situation. I was scheduled to be on the antibiotics for two weeks, but I felt fine after being in the hospital for only a few days. They wanted to keep me in the hospital for the full two weeks to be sure there were no more complications. I understood and appreciated their concern, especially given how sick I had been before we came back in to the hospital. I think the serious nature of the Meningitis also had them concerned for my safety. It was comforting to have them be so worried about me, but I was going nuts being in the hospital full time and only being treated two hours out of every day. We needed to figure out a better solution. I felt like I was being held hostage, even though it was for my own good while the doctors felt like I was being unreasonable for wanting to go home when I hadn't finished my course of treatment. The conversations got a little heated a couple of times. I'm sure we all understood both sides of the disagreement, but that didn't make a resolution any easier to find.

I thought the solution seemed simple enough: just send me home with a prescription for some antibiotics and I'll be fine. The doctors said that solution wouldn't work because the best antibiotics for the treatment needed to be administered intravenously. I suggested that they just leave my IV in my arm and send me home with the antibiotics and I could do it at home. We could get a home visit nurse to come check in on me if it would make them feel better. They said that the medication was caustic to my veins and the IV needed to be changed every few days in order to prevent permanent damage to my veins. I was out of ideas. I was going to be stuck in the hospital for two solid weeks with nothing to do but wait twelve hours for my next treatment. Thankfully, the doctors came up with an idea. The eventual solution? I was to be fitted with a PICC (peripherally inserted central catheter) line. The PICC is a small tube that would be inserted in a vein in my arm that would wind its way to a spot near my heart. The large quantity of blood-flow near my heart would dilute the antibiotics quickly and cause no damage to my veins. It wasn't exactly my ideal solution, but I was satisfied as long as I got to go home.

We've had a couple of different discussions about my trypanophobia (fear of needles) now. The insertion procedure of the PICC line was straight out of the darkest corners of that fear in my mind. I was wheeled on a gurney down to the radiology department for the PICC insertion because they needed to use ultrasound to ensure proper placement. There is a thin wire inside the PICC line to provide the stiffness needed for easy insertion. The wire is removed after the line has been placed correctly. It sounded to me suspiciously like using a wire coat hanger to run electrical wiring through a tight space in the wall. That wasn't a comforting thought. It wasn't actually like that at all. The team that inserted the line was excellent. They settled me into position on my gurney and got all of their equipment in place and ready to begin the insertion.

I was presented with a little bit of a quandary with the PICC insertion. I was very nervous, but I used my method of looking the other direction when they started to slide the line into my arm. I ended up looking right into the ultrasound monitor showing the PICC beginning its journey along the inside of my vein. Not good; not good at all. Nausea and dizziness instantly swept over me and I began to panic. I tore my eyes away from the monitor in a desperate attempt to not have a breakdown on the gurney, which brought my eyes straight back to the sight of the PICC line going into my arm. I completely freaked out. I closed my eyes and tried to stay calm and not get sick. I didn't really want to have another session of vomiting on hospital staff. After a couple of deep breaths, I squeaked out a request to the radiology team to see if they could put a towel or something over my eyes. They were happy to oblige as soon as they realized I was struggling and I got myself calmed down with their help. Once I was able to relax in my blind ignorance a little the rest of the process was very smooth.

They wheeled me back up to my room, through the now open airlock, and I got back into my bed. I never would have guessed that a hospital bed could be such an inviting place. After the terror of the PICC insertion process, I just wanted to curl up under my blankie and whimper for a little while. That didn't fit in the schedule for the evening, however. The head nurse came in and removed my IV, telling us that they would use the PICC line for the next couple of antibiotic treatments to be sure that it was working correctly. The nurses had Kay and I watch the process of administering the medication via the PICC both that evening and the next morning to give us an idea of what was involved.

I was released from the hospital the next evening with a delivery of medication and IV equipment scheduled at home and an appointment with the home nurse set up to teach me how to use the PICC line at home for the next morning.

When we got home that night, our friends, Rick and Cindy (who had shoveled the gravel), called and offered to come over to visit and bring pizza. It was great to be able to talk about some of the crazy things that had been happening with friends. Adding pizza to the mix just made it even better. Cindy had also made us a fantastic chicken enchilada casserole that we enjoyed for several days afterward without having to do any major meal fixing. I had never tasted better chicken enchiladas!

Bogey, Bill, and Betty had done fine at the house with Pat while we were gone. Bogey loves Pat, and Bill's silly antics along with Betty's buck teeth provided plenty of entertainment while we were gone. The time also allowed my sister to discover the joys of living with greyhounds. She had called us at the hospital at one point to ask if the dogs were really supposed to sleep that much. We explained that they were just couch potatoes even though they could reach speeds over 40mph when necessary. Pat had ended up texting pictures of Bill sprawled out on the sofa in the family room to all her friends. She just wasn't sure what to make of Betty's princess-like attitude, given the dental challenges that dog is stuck with. Poor Betty is a sweetie, but has some genuinely snarled up buck teeth. We were pleased that Pat had such a good time with the dogs.

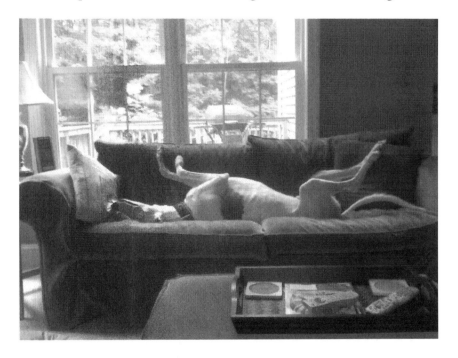

I was glad to be back home again even if I was a little creeped out by the PICC line that had allowed me the flexibility to be away from the hospital. Describing the feeling that looking at the PICC sticking out of my arm gave me is problematic. It didn't elicit the sheer terror that hypodermic needles did, but it produced a mild panic if I looked at it for too long or concentrated on the point where it entered my skin. The possibility of it getting caught on something and getting ripped out of my arm wasn't terribly comforting, either. The whole subject was just kind of gross.

The home visit nurse came to the house the next morning and showed me how to clean, prepare, and hook up the line to the antibiotics. The process involved cleaning the PICC fitting with an alcohol wipe, flushing the line with a 10cc pre-measured saline syringe, hanging the bag of antibiotics on an IV pole, and connecting the line from the bag to the PICC fitting. About thirty minutes later, when the antibiotic bag was empty, the PICC got disconnected from the bag line, cleaned again with an alcohol wipe, flushed out with another saline syringe, and flushed a second time with an anti-coagulant to ensure that the PICC line did not clog. Yeesh. The whole process took about 45 minutes and was to be done every twelve hours.

There was an odd thing that happened each time with the saline flush that the nurse asked me if I noticed. She asked if I could taste the saline. I didn't really understand what she was talking about, but I did notice that all this stuff smelled weird. It turned out that I experienced the saline as an odd smell instead of tasting it. Every time the line got flushed with the saline, I got a strange antiseptic smell in my nose. My questions to Kay about the smell elicited that familiar blank "what the hell are you talking about?" stare from her. I kept badgering her about the odd smell. How could she not smell it when it was so strong? She assured me that it was something that only I could smell. That was when I realized that somehow having the saline flushed into my bloodstream produced an odor to me. I don't really want to know how that might happen; some questions are just better left unexplored.

I ran into an issue when I tried to do the process myself because the PICC line ended just above my left wrist. That meant I couldn't use my left hand, but connecting the fittings was almost impossible to do with only one hand. Kay and I had to work out a schedule in the morning where she would do the first several steps and get the antibiotics hooked up just after we woke up and then go get ready for work while the bag emptied into my arm. Then she would flush the line just before she left for work. It wasn't quite as inconvenient in the evening since we could just sit and watch television for the thirty minutes it took for the bag to empty.

The PICC line procedure is just one more instance that shows the importance of having friends or family be involved in the recovery process. Hopefully, Meningitis treatment isn't something very many Acoustic Neuroma patients end up dealing with, but it demonstrates again how many people I counted on while I was getting better. There is just no way that I could have managed all the steps involved each time without help.

The home visit nurse returned half-way through the week to be sure things were going well. She was also available any time I had any questions or concerns, which was comforting. Thankfully, nothing came up.

Since I was feeling so much better, we started to go out in public more often again even while I still had the PICC. That provided no end of entertainment for me showing it to people and explaining how far up into my body it went. I was like a nine year old boy grossing out the other kids on the playground by eating worms. It was a nice distraction and diversion for me, and Kay was thrilled to have me feeling good enough to go out more. I'm not sure that our friends were quite as thrilled with me pointing out the nuances of my new medical appendage, but they were pretty patient with me.

The home nurse returned for my last antibiotic treatment so that she could remove the PICC line for me. My experience during my first hospital stay with the Foley catheter made me a little leery about removing this type of catheter. I asked the nurse about the process, and she told me that she would just pull it out gently. She assured me that it would not hurt. I still gag a little about the concept of pulling that line out of my arm, even though years have passed. I predictably turned my head and looked out the window and noticed a light pressure as she began pulling the tube out but nothing painful. I immediately made the mistake of looking at the line right after she removed it. Yuck. It was disgusting.

Now that I had survived my Meningitis infection, maybe things could get back to normal.

Part 4 – Moving Forward

13 – THE NEW NORMAL

Once we had the Meningitis out of the way, my recovery from the surgery could really get back on track to where it should have been weeks before. And it did. But things were different now. Lucky for me, I had a little bit of warning. I had several enlightening conversations with two people when we first found out about the tumor. Their advice was priceless as I started to put my life back together.

The first person that I had those conversations with was with my sister, Pat. Pat had been involved in an accident with a plate glass window in her mid-teens that had almost severed her left arm. The injuries left her with limited use of her left hand. It was Pat who told me about what she referred to as "the new normal." Things were going to be different now, and I was going to have to adapt to the changes as best I could.

The first, and most obvious, change was my face. I looked like a stroke victim. The right side of my face looked perfectly normal while the left side drooped uncontrollably. The doctors had assured me that things would start to move again in three to six months, but I was stuck with droopy for the time being. People stare. Some people even point and whisper. Great. But there wasn't anything I could do about it. I just ignored them the best I could, though I did grumble a little a couple of times at a guy in the hardware store who followed me around to stare at me. I don't know if he thought that I was some sort of idiot or what. I really felt like dressing him down in the middle of the store. It would have been fun to question his parentage and make some unkind comparisons between him and the more intelligent species on the planet- like some sort of garden slug. But while that might make me feel better, it wasn't going to change the fact that I looked different. Different always gets attention. I just let it go and got out of the store.

It still was difficult to look at myself in the mirror every day even though I knew it would get better. I hadn't really understood what "temporary paralysis" would entail, so there was no way for me to really prepare myself for this. Maybe my discussions about a lack of emotional preparation will help convince others that they should spend a little more time getting ready for a situation like mine. I don't think any description can prepare you for the realities of things, but maybe my frustrations can at least serve as a warning to get everyone thinking about their own new normal when something strikes out of the blue. What causes someone to experience their new normal doesn't really matter, it could be the loss of a loved one or a child starting a new school after a move. It just comes down to coping around whatever preparation you were able to make.

I realized right away that I needed to find some things to do that weren't affected by what my face looked like. Things where it just wouldn't matter. Remember the couple of references I made to bicycling? And the century ride I had set as my goal? My wife had been kind enough to purchase a new road bike for me after my surgery. Unfortunately, I had been so sick after the surgery and while I had Meningitis that I hadn't been able to ride it much.

The bike turned out to be just the answer I was looking for once I started to feel better. My bike never cared what my face looked like. It just felt fast and fun. I would ride it as far as my weak body could go and my bike never stared at me or pointed and whispered. All my bike wanted to do was get out on the road and ride. We spent a lot of time together in those autumn months. I ended up developing an interesting relationship with that bike while we were putting in the miles. It was my escape hatch; my pressure release valve. As my body got stronger, I kept racking up more and more miles. I developed a fun habit of using Google Maps to show me the road view of where I might be if I had just started riding from home and let my miles add up. I'd imagine myself riding through the mountains of West Virginia, then on into the old oil fields of Pennsylvania, and beyond. I loved the freedom that the bike gave me from the constant reminders of my situation. I could go out for a few hours and ride until I was exhausted, all the while just concentrating on riding. I didn't ever have to occupy my thoughts with anything else while I was out there. I could just be in the zone and pedal. The only time we didn't ride was in the rain due to the risk of a fall. But my bike and I weren't scared of wind or cold or snow, there wasn't much that could stop us. We even set out to conquer all the toughest hills in our area together. The right side of my face almost always had a smile on it at the end of a good ride, whether the left side of my mouth could participate or not.

I would really suggest to anybody working through a tough situation to find a hobby or an activity that doesn't care "what your face looks like." If it works towards the goal you have set for your recovery, super. If not, no big deal. This is really just emotional therapy more than anything else. Things will get better, but you can't just sit around and feel sorry for yourself and eat cookies until they do. I had this feeling inside that I had survived something incredible, that I had risen above something that tried to get me down. The miles on the bike let me express that in a healthy and constructive way. I realize that the anthropomorphism that helped me build a relationship with my bicycle might seem odd, but it really helped me to have a cycling partner that was always what I wanted. Being a figment of my imagination allowed the bike to always push when I needed pushing and to give in just at the right time and agree that it was time to head home.

Bogey didn't care what my face looked like, either. He was my pal whether I had my eye taped shut and was drooling out the left side of my mouth or not, and no matter that I couldn't smile or frown. He was always glad to spend time with me. Even though my wife and family and friends were all making every effort to not make me feel self-conscious about what I looked like, it was still a huge comfort to have Bogey do so without even having to think about it. We were buddies as far as he was concerned, just like always. Bogey had come to us as a foster dog after the young man in his family went to college and he had become very depressed. I had filled the role of "boy" to Bogey right away. Every dog needs a boy or girl in his life, right? It was a role that needed to be filled in his situation, and I was just the right person to fill it. We had been the best of pals ever since. It was so comforting to know that I hadn't changed in Bogey's eyes- I was just Daddy. On the days where my new normal was a real challenge, being with my little buddy, who thought that everything was just like it always had been, was priceless.

I really felt like something was missing during this phase of my recovery, though. I felt depressed sometimes. The bike was a great help, but I could only ride so far. Given how weak I still was physically, that wasn't incredibly far. Plus, I had been counting on so many of my friends, family, and doctors for support that I felt like I had become completely dependent on others. I could not thank all of those people enough for the kindness and support they showed me, but I felt like something really obvious was missing. I was saved by our greyhound rescue group.

We had taken some time off from our role as a foster home with the local greyhound rescue group to give me some recovery time. The foster coordinator with the Greyt Expectations called me in October to see if I felt up to having a couple of dogs foster with us. These two dogs had been returned to the group by their family because of a financial crisis. Let's be honest, a financial crisis was not uncommon in 2009. Enter Throttle and Clutch. Both dogs were underweight, lethargic, hadn't had regular vet care recently, and were obviously just sad after the separation from their family. They were in need of some love and attention.

Those two boys were just like Bogey in that they could not care less about what my face looked like. All they cared about was me (and Kay) loving them and taking good care of them. Being "Uncle Chris" to those two was a very important part of my emotional recovery at that point. Throttle, Clutch, and I all got ourselves better over the next couple of months, both physically and emotionally. Clutch got over most of his fears and issues and went back to being the love machine that I'm sure he had always been before. Throttle's personality came out a little more each day until he became a clown that performed in a greyhound suit. He was a nut. He had embraced his new normal with both paws. Kay discovered just how much his personality had blossomed out of his depression one day when she was working out. Kay was doing some yoga exercises on the floor of our family room. She was lying on her back on the floor doing whichever yoga thing when Throttle just couldn't stand it anymore- exercising just looked like too much fun! He got on the floor in a mirror image of Kay with his head touching hers and rolled onto his back. He wriggled out some doggy yoga to the point that Kay was laughing too hard to continue. He looked downright disappointed that she stopped; she figured he would have kept wriggling away as her yoga partner until he collapsed from exhaustion.

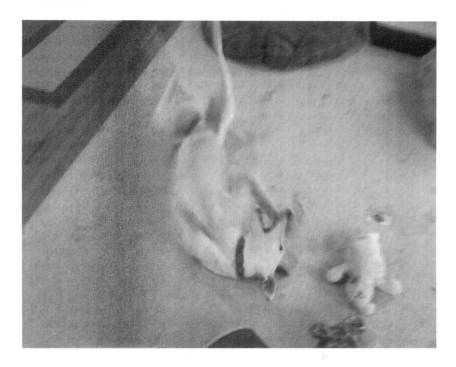

The important thing was that both boys were happy. That made me happy. Throttle and Clutch accepted their new situation and moved forward as best they could. They were such great examples to me and had done an amazing job of making me feel loved and wanted without a care in the world what my face looked like. They each went on to be adopted into their forever homes and I continued on with my recovery. The foster coordinator from the greyhound group had retired from a long career as a nurse. I think maybe there was some nursing going on for me as well as finding a soft landing spot for Throttle and Clutch. Thanks Cindy.

I realize that there are a lot of stories that have been told over the years about relationships like those I developed with Throttle and Clutch. It's the stereotypical story about the little girl who walks with crutches and ends up caring for the horse with leg broken so badly that everyone wanted to just shoot it. In the end, both the girl and the horse are able to run around and play together. It sounds just a little too storybook. But in my case, not only did it happen, those dogs are both off living happy lives thanks in part to the care they received while they were helping me deal with my issues. I've moved on in life as well, albeit a little different than it was before. But things were definitely better for me because of the friendship Throttle and Clutch gave without discrimination or hesitation. Among all the sweet dogs that have fostered with us over the years, those two hold a special spot in my heart because of the emotional growth we shared.

That happy little story brings us straight back to the new normal that I was learning to deal with. The surgery took what was left of the hearing in my left ear. I was now completely deaf in that ear. I knew going into the surgery that this would happen, but it was still very distracting. I couldn't tell where sounds were coming from. Your ears work together to help pinpoint sounds in three-dimensional space. Being deaf in one ear is like covering up one eye- you don't have any depth perception. If someone called my name, I would have to look all around me to find someone who looked like they might be expecting an answer from me. I could hear them just fine. I just couldn't tell where they were. There were several instances where this happened to me. One was on a group bike ride when a large group of riders was stopped at a red light. I recognized the voice of a friend who called my name and I just looked around with a stupid expression on my face. My friend finally called my name and told me where to look and I found her. I think it probably looked like the whole thing was some ridiculous act to the other riders stopped there, but without her guiding my gaze with "a little more to the right, now stop," I never would have found her.

This new reality meant that I needed to adapt. Fast. Otherwise I was going to get hurt. I learned that I was safest walking in a parking lot keeping all the parked cars on my left. That meant any sound that I heard of a moving car was most likely on my right side. And even if it was on my left, the car was probably just pulling out of a parking spot and wasn't moving fast enough to hit me very hard. Crossing aisles in parking lots to get to the correct side for me drives my wife crazy, but she gave up trying to convince me otherwise and now just crosses with me. Another adaptation I made was putting a mirror on my bicycle. I'm sure I look silly to other riders by having a rear-view mirror on my carbon fiber bicycle, but it has become a necessity at this point. Vehicle law dictates that bicycles stay as far right as possible on a road without a shoulder. That leaves my deaf ear facing traffic and leaves me with the difficult task of trying to identify where a car that I hear might be. Sometimes I don't hear a car until it is already beside me. Not good. The mirror shows me a little movement that catches my eye, and leaves me time to be sure I'm in a safe spot for the car to pass.

I found inspiration to help deal with my Single Sided Deafness on day in a random internet browsing session. I found a man in the UK who was legally blind, yet training for an ultra-marathon. He could barely distinguish between light and dark, yet he was going to run a race that covered one-hundred miles in a single day. I was fascinated. Here was someone who had a far more difficult sensory deprivation than I did, but he was still attempting to do something extraordinary. He posted a movie one day on his Blog that he had taken with his cellphone showing his training route. He narrated for the audience, telling us what he clues to his environment he was using to navigate- sounds, changes in footing, and shadows. The fact that he could navigate his running route with only subtle changes in terrain under his feet, shadows from things overhead, and the ambient sound was incredible. I decided right then that if this guy could run with almost no vision, I could do whatever I wanted on that bike. And it didn't matter whether I had an ugly mirror on my cool bike or not, I just needed to get out there and ride.

Being deaf in one ear also makes the movie going experience a little less exciting. All that cool 7.1 digital audio that they use in new movies? It's completely lost on me. I no longer have any concept of surround sound at all. Things just get louder and softer. I got a good laugh one day from a website I happened upon when I was researching Single Sided Deafness. There was a quote about how surround sound was for other people. And they were absolutely right.

For those of us affected by it, there are several good options for helping deal with Single Sided Deafness (SSD). And more appear in the marketplace every year. There are several different brands and levels of CROSS hearing aids. The CROSS systems use a hearing aid on the deaf side with a microphone that transmits sound from that side to another hearing aid in the good ear, either wired or wireless. The downside is having to wear a hearing aid in your good ear.

Most of the rest of the options for SSD that I have seen involve bone conduction. Bone conduction uses the ability of the skull to transfer sound via vibration. One device, called a BAHA unit, uses a surgically implanted titanium stud in your skull behind the deaf ear. There is a microphone unit that snaps onto the stud behind your ear with an oscillator that vibrates the stud, sending vibrations through your skull to the good ear. Another option uses a unit that looks very much like a normal behind-the-ear (BTE) hearing aid, but with a much deeper part that goes into the ear. The part of the unit in the ear has a tiny oscillator that vibrates the bones deep in the ear canal, thus sending vibrations through the skull to the hearing ear. I tried one of these units with some success. I found that I could pinpoint sounds quite well with it. The unit was not as comfortable as I had hoped. There is a third option that utilizes a BTE type device on the deaf ear and sends a wireless signal to an oscillation unit that clamps to your teeth on the hearing side and sends vibrations to the good ear.

The different options all have some drawbacks, mostly involving comfort. They vary significantly in price, though most should be at least partially covered by insurance. For my fellow AN'ers, I would suggest a thorough internet search in order to find all the options out there. This is a market that will continue to grow with new products being approved frequently by the FDA. I don't think that many doctors or hearing specialists will be well informed about all the latest products, so it will be up to the patient to ask the right questions. But however you try to work with it, deafness is often, though not always, part of the new normal for us.

My search for a the bone conduction hearing-aid took me to the only audiologist in the DC area that I could find with any experience with them. She went through her normal examination process, which I understood, but then she wanted to give me a standard hearing test. I gave her a lopsided smile and explained that the surgery had taken all of my hearing in my left ear. I even showed her the scar and explained about my facial nerve. She said she still wanted to do a hearing test. Okie-dokie! So we did a hearing test. I felt a little silly sitting in a sound-proof booth with headphones on raising only my right hand, but what was I supposed to do? I understood her desire to do the test, even though I was pretty certain what the results would be. The chart for my right ear looked just like every other recent hearing test I had been through over the last year or so. The chart for my left ear, however, was flat-line. Not a single response. The audiologist realized that I wasn't kidding about being stone deaf on that side and got me fit for the hearing aid.

My mouth was another new reality to get used to. The left side of my mouth didn't always react the way I thought it would in those first few months. It was downright unpredictable. Food might fall out of my mouth while I was eating, which was sometimes very embarrassing in public. Again, my wife and friends would come to the rescue. No, they didn't throw errant food back in, but they did politely ignore the fact that half of the mouthful of burrito that I was chewing just dropped out of the left side of my mouth and into my lap. I learned to warn people who were less aware of my situation that I didn't necessarily have full control of my mouth. I found that most people who were not experienced in my new normal just tended to keep their eyes averted when I was eating. I was OK with that; I gave them an "A" for effort.

Brushing my teeth continued to be an adventure. I got very good at leaning down directly over the sink to try to avoid making too much of a mess, and I discovered a method of rinsing that involved using my fingers to pinch the left side of my lips together. Straws still only worked on the right corner of my mouth. I had to slide any type of burger or sandwich into my mouth from right to left. Whistle? Nope, I was never going to whistle again. My acoustic guitar version of the Scorpion's "Wind of Change" would just never be the same. And I surely would never be able to whistle Dixie, not that a lack of Dixie was going much of a problem in my life.

Whistling was just another of those little things that I missed. I loved to play bad rock covers on my guitar that involved whistling, along with entertaining myself with old Eddie Murphy jokes about cologne, or just whistling a happy little tune once in a while. Would my inability to whistle have some huge affect on my life? No, but having some of the little pleasures in life taken away was disappointing. I imagine that people who suffer from debilitating arthritis feel a similar disappointment. It's hard when the little things you enjoy become impossible. It feels like yet another gift has been taken from you without your permission. I still miss whistling a tune. Maybe I should get a harmonica.

A completely unforeseen challenge for my mouth came up when I tried calling our health insurance company to ask a couple of questions. They used a voice recognition program on their telephone system that didn't understand me because my mouth didn't work right. The system would ask me to read my insurance number to it, but I was completely unintelligible to the machine. It kept telling me to try again or that it hadn't understood. Because the policy number involved letters as well as numbers, there was no way to punch it in on the keypad. I just had to wait until the system transfered me to an operator to help me with my call. I didn't even have the excuse of an old and faded matchbook. I was really frustrated at first; I just didn't need one more damned thing reminding me of how screwed up my face was. A thought occurred to me as I sat down feeling angry about it. It was a good challenge. I could make talking to the stupid health insurance phone machine a new goal! I just put it on a back burner in my mind to simmer for a while.

The new realities that I had to work around with my eye were no fun in those first few months either. Several functions in and around the eye depend on that facial nerve that was not working at that particular point in time. The blink process depends on the facial nerve, as do normal tear production and sinus function. My left eye drove me crazy. I couldn't close it, so it didn't blink on its own. Add a lack of tear production to a lack of blinking and you end up with a very dry and irritated eye. I used artificial tear drops and ointments to keep the eye lubricated, but I still had to blink the eye manually using a finger to pull the lid down. At night it was usually most comfortable if I just taped it closed, which produced more depressed feelings. How pathetic was I that I just gave up and taped my eye closed at night? Who can't close their stupid eye? The frustration was palpable some days. On the days that nothing else worked to comfort my eye, I would resort to using an eye ointment. It provided a lot of comfort to my eye, but it completely blurred the vision in that eye. So there I'd be with vision in only one eye and hearing in only one ear. I suppose I was was lucky that I didn't have a penchant for dodge-ball. I would have been a sitting duck. Having no tears meant I had to shampoo my hair with one hand while the other hand held my eyelid closed as tightly as possible. The lack of facial nerve signals made my sinuses run at weird times on just the left side. There was truly nothing more gratifying than stopping at a stop sign on a bike ride with friends to discover that the left side of your nose was running profusely. Not both sides, just that left side since the sinuses were confused given the damage to the facial nerve.

Even the normal things about the eye that hadn't been affected by the surgery were problematic. I found some really good eye drops, but they disappeared very quickly down the ducts that the eye uses normally to drain tears. I asked my eye doctor about it when I went to get new glasses. Without any tear production, I couldn't wear contact lenses anymore so I had to revert back to eyeglasses. My optometrist had a great solution for me to fix the drain duct issue. He put in a Punctal Plug, which sealed off the natural drain in my lower eyelid and allowed the eye drops to stay in place longer and increase my comfort level. Just one more creepy thing to fix the side effects of the surgery.

There was nothing easy in my new normal. Even the simple process of picking out frames for my new eyeglasses was a challenge since the hole in my skull was right where the bow of the glasses would sit. I had to find a pair that could be adjusted to still fit straight even with the bow poking into the hole in my skull.

The second person I had conversations with when I first found out about the surgery was with our friend, Peter. He had a very invasive heart surgery a couple of years before I was diagnosed with my Acoustic Neuroma. He said his recovery had been really frustrating because he had tried to do too much, too soon. His advice to me was to understand that a full recovery was going to take at least as long as the longest predictions by any doctor or therapist. Or maybe even longer. He was very clear that I needed to just be patient and let things progress naturally. It was great advice that I probably should have paid more heed to right after my surgery. I definitely paid more attention after my Meningitis treatment. I only did what I was comfortable with. If I got tired, I went and got some rest and came back to the activity later. I really do learn these lessons eventually.

Working with Peter's theory on the predictions of medical professionals, my face didn't show any sign of movement for the full six months. Then one day something felt a little different.

14 – PHYSICAL THERAPY

Dr. Kim told me when I left the hospital back in July that I could start physical therapy on my face as soon as there was movement on the left side. He and Dr. Jean had assured me the paralysis was temporary, since they had tested the facial nerve during the surgery and it showed good conductivity. For the next six months, I would occasionally put a finger on the left side of my mouth or cheek and try to smile. One night just after Christmas- almost six months to the day- I felt my face move. It wasn't much movement, but it was the first time I had felt it move since July. I was ecstatic. I went to show Kay and she agreed that it was moving just a tiny little bit. She was a little less excited about it than I was since the movement could barely be seen, but it was definitely there. I called Dr. Kim early the next morning and he got me set up to begin physical therapy. I called several local therapy practices and found one with a therapist who had experience working with patients with facial paralysis.

My therapist, Danielle, was great. My initial interview and testing with her obviously showed only that tiny little movement my wife and I had seen the week before, but she wasn't put off by that at all. She put together a battery of exercises for me to practice all the movements I would need. During our appointments, I would work on each of those exercises so that Danielle could see what progress I had made since our last appointment. It was slow progress, but she always had a smile (with both sides of her mouth) for me as we worked to improve the range of motion and muscle strength. She also started me on electrical muscle stimulation. Yep, that's just what it sounds like. You've seen or heard of the high school biology experiments that make a frog leg twitch by introducing an electrical current to muscles, right? Same idea. Danielle would hook up electrodes to two places on my face, then low voltage electricity would pulse through at intervals while I practiced an exercise that used those muscles. It was not a pleasant process, but my face kept getting more movement so I didn't complain. OK, I didn't complain too much. But every time I felt grumpy about being shocked over and over again, I'd think about how much better my face was going to be when we finished up therapy!

My therapy exercises included an embarrassing collection of opening my mouth as wide as I could, paying special attention to show my teeth, along with pucker up, smile, frown, and flare my nostrils. Who ever thought that flaring your nostrils would become a goal in life? Danielle and I must have looked completely absurd making all these faces at each other. We could have been the star attraction in a bad mime theater.

I was in physical therapy for about three months during which time my facial movement got much better. I could close my left eye, at first only in tandem with my right eye and only then with a lot of concentration. Later I got to the point where I could close them each on their own. The little successes were the most rewarding. When I first started to get movement back in my left eyelid, I would squeeze both eyes shut as tightly as possible. Obviously my right eye would close tightly, but the left one took time and practice. I remember being in the car with Kay at a stoplight one day showing her my "new" skill of being able to close both eyes. She tried to be patient with me, since the left one still didn't close quite all the way, but I was so excited about it that I don't think she had the heart to say too much. When I finally got the left eye to close completely, I felt like I had just topped Everest. It was such a feeling of accomplishment for me. Then I realized how excited I was to be staring at myself in the mirror and closing my eyes. My right eye offered a couple of tears of consolation, though the left one didn't have any tears to give. This was such a long and frustrating process.

One of the things I did to practice my eye closing was to alternate closing each eye like the old railroad crossing lights. I was so delighted with myself when I got it working right that I went to show Kay. It sounds like I was a kid with a coloring book that went to show Mommy every time I finished a small section of the picture, doesn't it? I guess it really was kind of like that. She confided in me that she couldn't alternate closing her eyes, even with full control over her face. That made me feel better.

By the time my three months of therapy was over, my face had enough structure and strength that if you saw me in public you'd never notice that I was different. I considered it success. I wished I could find the guy that had done all the staring in the hardware store that day several months before to show him how far I'd come. Then I realized how pathetic that feeling of resentment was. I had to rise above stuff like that and just move forward.

In the end, there was still a new normal for my face. I'd say that I have about 70% movement back. That's probably a little optimistic, but I'm sticking to it. In reality, I probably have less than 50% of the movement back. I'll never be able to move my left eyebrow again, which marked a dramatic improvement in my John Belushi impression. As I mentioned before, I won't ever whistle again, nor will the left side of my mouth ever participate much in smiling again. But my tear production came back for the most part, I could use a straw, I could brush my teeth without having to use my fingers (as long as I was careful), and food didn't fall out of my mouth as a general rule. It wasn't the end result I might have hoped for, but I try not to complain. I make an effort not to dwell on it, but I do sometimes anyway.

I am acutely self conscious of the way my face looks. I know that it doesn't appear different at first glance to people, but I am always thinking about how it comes across. I noticed one day when a friend was sharing some group pictures that he had taken from a night out to dinner with a group, that the difference in my face was obvious in the photos. I spent weeks after that in front of the mirror trying to memorize the feeling of the muscles around my mouth that most closely resembled my mouth being straight. It didn't really work. The muscles just don't do that anymore, but I can at least get it to not look droopy. Too vain? No way!

I have finally found that I just make a little effort and call it good enough. It's never going to be perfect again. Hell, I wasn't even very good at smiling before I had the surgery. Kay framed a photo of the two of us attending her brother's wedding just because we both look good and I've got an actual smile on my face. Otherwise, the best you usually got from me was a happy showing of my teeth.

Maybe my smile isn't such a big loss after all. It does put me into a very specific club online where the emoticon: :-/ means that I'm smiling. That's exactly what my face looks like if I smile without thinking.

I was finally able to call our health insurance company's automated phone answering system and get the voice recognition software to understand me. I called back a couple of times just to be sure, but I would hang up before being connected to an agent so as not to waste anyone's time. Finally, I called back one last time and talked to a customer service agent just to share my happiness. I could tell that the agent wasn't sure what to think, but she told me that she was happy for me and that it was a bright spot in her day. I can see where having me call to tell you that I was excited to be understood by the voice recognition software would be far better than arguing with an angry customer over an insurance payment. I know I was excited about it.

There are a lot of little details in my new normal. Things you wouldn't think about but end up having an effect not only on me, but on the people around me. Because of the deafness, I had to learn where the best places for me to sit in a restaurant or at a table with a group. Restaurants, bars, and any other place with a lot of noise present significant difficulty. But I learned to keep as many of the people as possible on my right side. If I have the chance, I will always choose a left most corner of any table. My wife had to learn this as well so that we didn't have to have a committee meeting every time somebody asked her where we wanted to sit. Single Sided Deafness does provide a good excuse to ignore people on your left if you'd like. You just have to take their position at the table into account when you choose your seat. Maybe I shouldn't have shared that particular secret. Oops.

Check-out lanes in the grocery store are a nightmare for me. I'm not sure why, but most stores have their check-out lanes set up so that the checker is on your left side while you are going through the line. Check-out areas are usually noisy places, and I'm facing the wrong way, usually working with the credit card machine, when the clerk will ask me a question. I've learned that the question is most likely to be "will you need any assistance outside, sir?" or something similar. I just half-smile a little and tell them no, thank you, I'll be fine. That works great right up until I realize that they must have asked me something that makes that answer sound stupid, even though that answer will work for all sorts of questions they might ask. But if it happened to be a question about whether I had the day off work, or if I was going to cheer for the Baltimore Ravens or the Washington Redskins this Sunday, I looked like an idiot. New normal when it comes to being deaf on one side? Sometimes you look like a moron. I guess it just comes with the territory.

There are some upsides to being deaf on one side. I usually sleep with my good ear down to the pillow so I don't hear much ambient noise, allowing me to sleep like the dead. I don't have to drag around a set of stereo earbuds to listen to music. I have a single that uses a stereo plug; several options of them are available online. I do make sure to take better care of the hearing in my right ear than I used to. If I lose the hearing in that side, then I'm just deaf. I wear an earplug pretty often in my good ear when I'm doing any lawn mowing or other loud activity.

But Kay and I aren't the only ones who had to adjust to my new situation. This whole process presented a challenge for my hair stylist and the other salon staff at the place where I get my hair cut. My stylist, Ami, is great. We always had a lot of fun when I got my hair cut before I was diagnosed with my tumor. I went to see her a few days before the surgery to get my hair cut short so there wouldn't be such a huge difference when the doctors shaved part of my head. I figured that I wouldn't be able to get a haircut for a while, so short hair would be a good plan no matter.

The realities of the surgery and its aftermath created some new challenges for Ami. After I had gotten over the Meningitis, I really needed a haircut. It had been over a month since I had my pre-surgical short cut. I still had my sutures in, and my face was droopy which made me nervous about how I would be received at the salon, but the mop on my head had to get trimmed whether people stared at me or not. I should have known better than to think anyone would stare, since the whole crew at Scalped Salon & Spa are awesome. All the staff who knew me stopped over to say hello, and not a single person treated me any different from normal even though I looked very different. I'm not sure if they're all just great people, or if they get that from Margaret, the owner. I'm sure it's a combination of both. They are a fantastic group of people. It was a nice boost to my confidence to have a bunch of nice looking ladies smile and ask how

I was doing without looking at me like I was some sort of freak show.

Ami created the gold standard for great treatment at the salon on that first visit back after the surgery. She was a little put off by the sutures at first. She was very careful around them when she washed my hair, then asked me if I was sure I really wanted her to cut around them. Yes, please cut this mop off my head! Imagine the courage it took for her to cut my hair so near my surgical site. She was working with razor sharp scissors and electric clippers around the entry point where I had brain surgery. I'm sure that is something they don't teach in cosmetology or barber school. She did a great job.

Poor Ami was still hesitant even after my sutures had been removed. She wanted to be absolutely sure that she didn't injure me or accidentally cause me any pain, which I appreciated. I probably didn't help the matter by making her feel around the edges of the hole in my skull, but I just couldn't help myself. I figured that it would be good for her to understand what was under the scar, though I don't think she'd agree. It seemed to me that running a finger around the rim of the opening in my skull would be a great tactile reinforcement of what she saw, but I think poor Ami could have lived to a ripe old age and died a happy grandmother without ever feeling like she had missed out on anything by not feeling the hole in my head. Ami was very attentive to the entirety of my new normal, making sure that we didn't get any hair in my eye that wouldn't close yet, and she was extra careful around the scar area. She had to learn to adapt to me being deaf, too. She has learned not to talk to me if there are clippers or a hairdryer on my hearing side. We even had to have a bone conduction lesson so that she understood that having the clippers in contact with my skull on the deaf side is almost the same as holding them in front of my good ear. I will not be able to hear any conversation while they are in contact. Is any of this a big deal? No, of course not. But it's just one more way someone around me has had to change their thinking to work around my new situation.

15 – MOVING ON

My Acoustic Neuroma has been a life changing event for me. Moving on was not a simple thing, but I feel like I have persevered and have gotten back to living my life within the new boundaries that I was presented.

I achieved my goal of riding one hundred miles on my bicycle by completing the Seagull Century in October of 2010. That goal had kept me going for over a year from those early days in my hospital bed. It gave me reason to get off my butt and leave the house in the months that followed and helped me get my weakened body stronger a little bit at a time. Planning from the outset to wait at least a year to complete it was a smart thing because it gave me a nice easy path to reach my goal. This photo shows me crossing the finish line on that October day:

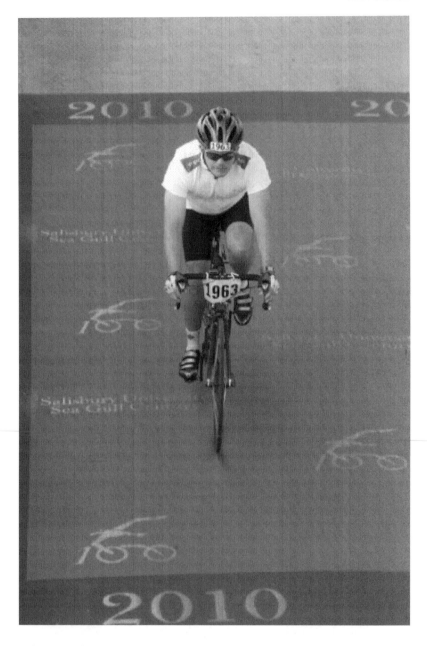

I have talked endlessly about how important family and friends are in dealing with my tumor and recovery. The century ride was just another example of how powerful those relationships were. All my friends knew about my goal of completing that ride, and they showed up in force to support me. One of my friends made an announcement at an awards banquet in January that she was going to ride those one-hundred miles with me in October no matter what. She was true to her word and was there for the ride along with a bunch of my other friends. About a dozen of them did the ride, while several others joined my wife as support and photo crew. Obviously they were there to enjoy the ride and the camaraderie with friends as well as supporting me, but they could have done that with any ride in the season. They were doing this particular ride as my friends, and it meant the world to me.

My family and friends supported me through every turn from the beginning of my journey right up to the very end. They offered their time, their expertise, and most of all their friendship to me in my time of need. I thanked them all over and over again, but it never feels like enough. How do you thank people for being willing to change your bandages for you? Or for not being annoyed when you make them feel the hole the doctors drilled in your skull? Or for making a four hour drive to ride one-hundred miles on a bicycle with you? I think the best way for me to say thank you is to keep living my new normal to its fullest. I will persevere. I will continue on. I will not give up. Thanks to them.

Finishing the bike ride turned into a renewed interest in physical fitness. I'm never going to be an Adonis figure carved out of stone, but I lost a significant amount of weight and continue to achieve new fitness goals.

The ordeal we went through was a wonderful reminder to my wife and me to keep on our life plan of making the best use of our best years. We are trying to not wait to do the things we want in life until it is too late. Having a brain tumor is a great reminder that things aren't always going to go the way you want them to. We have a solid set of plans and goals that we work towards every day regarding travel, entertainment, sailing, and other things we enjoy doing. Kay and I have met a lot of people over the years that scrimped and saved their entire lives to purchase their dream sailboat and do all the sailing they wanted in retirement. Only to have one of them fall ill, or face some other tragedy. Having a brain tumor in your mid-thirties is a great reminder to get out there and do the stuff you want to do. Now. Don't wait.

That wasn't the only reminder that my Acoustic Neuroma

provided. It was a good reminder for me to be thankful for the people who made my successful recovery possible. I thanked my surgical team repeatedly at every follow-up appointment. I thanked my friends and family for their continued support. And I took the time to write a nice thank you note to Dr. Glenn Marinelli and dropped it off at his office one day after my recovery. I wanted him to know that I was doing okay after the surgery. Dr. Marinelli tragically passed away just two years later. I obviously appreciate all that he did for me, and I'm grateful that I was able to thank him before he left us.

I think it is important to give back when you have been given a gift. I wouldn't ever consider having an Acoustic Neuroma a gift, but I think my positive long term recovery is definitely a gift. In order to give back where I could, I participated in social media and online discussion groups. I am always an advocate for an MRI any time someone has Acoustic Neuroma type symptoms. These all seemed like small things to me, but I couldn't think of a way to be more helpful until I was given an opportunity to help someone more directly.

I got a random call from my friend, Kim, one night. She had a lot of questions about the symptoms I had early on that led to the decision to get the MRI that found the tumor. She was having almost identical symptoms. We talked for a long time that night on the phone about all the things that had happened to me. I couldn't believe it. Her symptoms sounded just like mine. She went back to her doctors armed with a little more information that helped get the right answers to questions. She had an Acoustic Neuroma. So much for them being incredibly rare. She called me a couple of days later to give me the news. I just stood in our kitchen, leaning against the counter in front of the sink, my "Gould" spot, and shook my head while I listened. I felt terrible for her.

I realized that I had been given a unique opportunity to provide support. We talked on the telephone several times and I gave her all the information I could think of. She ended up having her surgery at Georgetown performed by Dr. Kim and Dr. Jean. I hoped that my experience would help Kim and her family prepare as much as possible for the difficult months ahead. I was so relieved when we got the news that her surgery had been successful! I made sure to do all the things that I had found so kind when people were supporting me. I told Kim's family to call me if they had any questions about anything. I sent flowers and a teddy bear to her in the hospital. I went to visit her when she got out of the hospital and took along a couple of home-made meals that were easily reheated. Who doesn't love home-made Mac & Cheese?

The point of this is not that I'm a great guy, though you're welcome to think that about me if you like. I won't argue. The point is that helping out someone else was a fantastic way to continue my recovery while getting Kim started on the road to hers. The crooked smile that I saw the day I went to see Kim after she got out of the hospital was perfect. Her son and her dog were both on duty taking care of her, and the four of us sat and talked for about an hour until she started to get tired. Kim seemed like she had a much less eventful recovery than I did, thankfully.

Kim and I share a special bond since her surgery. Any time we see each other we sit down with my good right ear facing her good left ear and we just ignore everyone else and chat for a while. If people want to talk to us, we can make a theatrical switch so that our deaf ears face each other and make a show of ignoring each other while we talk to other people. I guess there are a few other benefits to being deaf on one side, especially when you have a friend to enjoy it with.

16 – FINAL THOUGHTS

I've described my physical recovery in great detail, but I've only touched on some of the emotions that went along with it. My emotional recovery has taken much longer than it took for my body to heal. I'm sure that's probably normal. It isn't something I advertise or let everyone see, but I think it's important that I share it with people who are affected by something similar to what I went through. I hope that it provides a little insight to family and friends so that they can look behind the curtain that is the half smile of someone who has dealt with Acoustic Neuroma. There is most likely some lingering anger, frustration, and sadness behind that curtain somewhere.

I was pretty upbeat during my initial hospital stay following the surgery. Obviously there were some troubling things that happened as well as some expected bad days. I was pretty happy that I had gotten that far. I'm willing to chalk a lot of the optimism up to large quantities of narcotics, but nobody ever said that painkillers couldn't have positive side effects while they were doing their job, right? I don't think where the optimism comes from is important. Even though the Meningitis wasn't much fun, things were OK once we got back on track towards recovery.

The dark days came later. I knew that I would lose my hearing and thought I was mentally prepared for it. Nope. Not by a long shot. As much as I joke about gossiping with my friend and getting spectacular sleep, I hate it. I hate having to crane my neck around to get my ear towards people talking to me. Having a conversation as a passenger in my wife's convertible is all but impossible; I might as well read a book. Then there's the music. I studied music in school. I have a music degree. I have played music all of my life. Then I lost half of my hearing and ended up with a mouth that doesn't work right. Being deaf in one ear takes away some of the nuance of the sounds that my guitar makes. It leaves my senses overpowered on my right side and clueless about what's going on over to the left. Turning my head while I play my guitar almost has a Doppler effect, the sound changes so much. It's all very frustrating. It's a good thing that I hadn't played my trombone much over the past several years, since my mouth being messed up means I'll never play it again.

Beethoven? Yes, you're absolutely right. He was mostly deaf. Actually, he used to stick his head on the piano in order to take advantage of the bone conduction we talked about earlier. And Beethoven did write some wonderful music after his hearing loss, but he was miserable. My loss of hearing doesn't make me miserable, per say, but it certainly does make me frustrated.

Remember the photo I showed you from just before I went in for surgery? I'm happy to explain why I hate that photo. That photo represents everything that my life was before. I was fat, ignorant, and happy. Why wouldn't I be? I didn't have the slightest clue what was about to happen to me. That's the last image I have of the left side of my mouth participating in a smile. It's the last time you could have called my name and I would have known immediately where to look. And it's the last time I felt whole. It was the end of my old normal.

Everything changed that day. Other people have major surgeries and it doesn't seem to have as much of an effect on them as mine did on me. I think they hide it just like I do. Something happened on that operating table that changed me forever. It wasn't an easy thing to figure out in the first year or so after. But I would manage in time and learn to cope. I would learn to make the best of it. I wonder sometimes, though, if other people that have had excessively long surgical procedures or suffered major trauma have felt that same change that I did from the surgery. Maybe someday I'll have to ask around, but I'm too frightened of the answers I might get for now.

There are scars that I will carry with me into the future. Some you can see clearly by looking at me, although the incision scar is hidden nicely under my hair, and some you can't see unless you look a little deeper. The paper towel dispensers that I despise are a good example. How many people do you know are terrified by the sounds associated with washing their hands? At least there aren't any more monsters on posters reminding people to wash up and use the paper towel machine.

I still harbor some anger at the nurse practitioner who thought hot showers and bowls of steaming water would cure my brain tumor. I thought about filing a lawsuit, but decided against it. I would have wanted them to revoke her license to practice, but the ensuing case would have most likely settled out of court and just raised malpractice insurance rates on competent professionals. That wouldn't help anyone at all, so I didn't bother. I'm thankful for the great medical professionals who helped me, and I'll let that be enough. I do hope that Karma makes a visit to that lady, though. It would make me feel better.

This is my new reality. That tumor would have killed me eventually had I not gotten it removed. It most likely wouldn't have even taken very long to do so, as big as it was. But I'm still here, and I've taken away a new outlook on life with a more adventurous spirit. My new perspective is allowing me to explore and embrace new things without fear. My new adventurous spirit doesn't include anything to do with needles, or probably skydiving. It does include just about anything else, though. Life changes, physical challenges, or even dealing with difficult people doesn't really scare me anymore. I guess even writing a book isn't frightening. I've always wanted to write a book, and now I have. I'm guessing it won't be my last.

My emotional recovery hasn't been fun or easy. It has been a been a long road with some dark and scary days, but the destination I've reached is a good one. I am moving forward as a more complete person with a better outlook on the future and no interest in dwelling on the past. My recovery will probably continue for the rest of my life as I conquer new things, fail miserably at others, and have one heck of a good time doing it all. I didn't end up with any spiritual insight or a religious awakening from my experiences, but I can understand where others might. I guess I ended up with a better view into myself; let's call it a personal awakening. I'm happy with that.

Diagnosis: Brain Tumor

17 – A LITTLE ADVICE

My story is not an instruction manual for anyone, nor should it ever be considered medical advice. So what do I hope you take away from it?

If you have an Acoustic Neuroma? I sympathize. That sucks. It really does. I hope that you and your doctors have caught it small enough that any procedure you have is a simple one. I hope that my story has armed you with information that might help make your journey a little easier. I cannot stress enough the importance of surrounding yourself with people who care about you. Let them help you with all this. Ask your health care professionals questions and do as much learning on your own as you can. Make sure you understand what is going to happen to you. Find the best doctors you can to treat your Acoustic Neuroma. Don't let your recovery get you down- there are a lot of people out there with long term effects from an Acoustic Neuroma who are doing all sorts of cool stuff. Set a goal to let yourself know that you're back. Then find a way to give back for all the kindness people have given you. Most important of all, I wish you good luck.

Are you a family member or loved one of an Acoustic Neuroma patient? I hope my story helps you to be a stronger member of the support crew. Go with the patient to appointments with doctors. Take notes to be sure a nervous patient doesn't miss anything. You can help with research and reading. In fact, you already are! I'm sure that if you've found my story, it isn't the first reading you've done. Try to take a few days off from work around any surgeries or treatments if you can. Or maybe you could work from home for a couple of days during their recovery? That would be great. I'm sure your loved one would really appreciate it.

Are you a friend or co-worker? Send a note or card. Go visit them in the hospital or when they get home. You can't imagine how good seeing a familiar face they weren't expecting will make them feel. Try to work within the bounds of their new normal. Do your best to remember things like which ear to talk to. It's no big deal if you forget, but it will be a huge help when you remember. Do you have any skills that could help after a surgery or other medical treatment? Are you a nurse? A good cook? Great with kids or pets? Help out if you can. Dealing with a brain tumor and its aftermath is plenty stressful without having to worry about the kids, dog, or what the family is going to eat for dinner tonight.

Are you someone who doesn't have any connections to Acoustic Neuroma at all? First, let me welcome to our little corner of the world. It's a pretty strange place sometimes. Here's how our initial conversation would probably go from my side. You've got a few questions? Pretty much everyone asks the same things on your side: *Yes, I had a brain tumor. No, it wasn't cancer. No, I had never heard of it before, either. Actually, somewhere in between one and two percent of the population have them. Thanks, I appreciate that- I'm pretty glad that I survived the experience, too!*

There are a lot of great awareness campaigns that go on all the time for medical conditions including breast cancer, AIDS, autism, and many others that have made the world more conscious of the plight of people affected by those things. It's wonderful that each of those conditions has been brought more acutely into the minds of people around the world. Acoustic Neuroma is one of the many medical conditions that doesn't have that type of public relations campaign. I hope if you are someone who doesn't have any relation to Acoustic Neuroma at all, that you will share your new knowledge with other people. It might just help a patient find his or her tumor a little earlier, which allow them to have many more treatment options than the ones that I was presented with due to the size of my tumor.

And a thought for everybody from my experience. Please try to refrain from any statement including the words, "lucky it's not cancer." Yes, Acoustic Neuroma patients are very lucky that the tumor isn't cancerous. You're right. Malignant brain tumors are a horrible thing for someone to be presented with. But imagine what a statement like that might feel like to somebody with an Acoustic Neuroma. They have a brain tumor. Some will eventually grow to a size that will maim, if not kill. There could be invasive brain surgery involved. Cancer is a heinous disease, as anyone who has been affected by it knows- my family included. But don't diminish the serious nature of the brain tumor diagnosis, OK? I know that cancer is a delicate topic in society today, but hopefully I have offered a little insight into how a seemingly friendly statement could be taken the wrong way.

18 – MY FATHER'S WISDOM

I'm going to leave you with the best advice my Father ever gave me. Years ago when I was dealing with what seemed like a crisis at the time he said, "Is this the worst thing that's ever happened to you?" No. "OK, then. If you lived through something worse, you'll live through this." It sounds sort of silly and trite when you first hear it. But I can tell you that having an Acoustic Neuroma is easily the worst thing that has ever happened to me. I lived through it. There aren't too many things out there that I can think of that would be worse than my experience with the tumor, so I should be pretty well set for a while. Parts of me have struggled along the way and I've had to work through some difficult places, but parts of me have thrived and I've challenged myself to new achievements. I don't really worry about much anymore in life. I just live every day like I want to. I wish you the best in doing the same.

ACOUSTIC NEUROMA RESOURCES

Acoustic Neuroma Association- www.Anausa.org

American Brain Tumor Association- www.Abta.org

The National Institutes of Health have a couple of informative websites:

www.ncbi.nlm.nih.gov/pubmedhealth/pmh0001782/

www.nlm.nih.gov/medlineplus/acousticneuroma.html

CaringBridge is a fantastic way to easily keep friends and family updated- www.caringbridge.org

There is an amazing Acoustic Neuroma group on Facebook- just search for "Acoustic Neuroma"

ABOUT THE AUTHOR

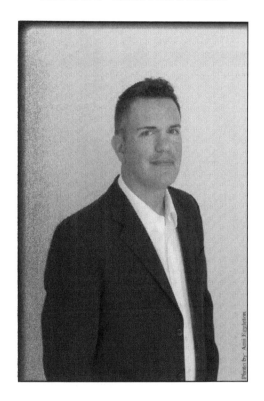

C. Michael Miller lives in Maryland with his wife, his greyhound, Bogey, and whichever foster dog might be in residence at the time. You might see him riding his bicycle, sailing on the Chesapeake Bay, or hear him playing his guitar in the cockpit after dinner. He is passionate about greyhound rescue.

You can find more information at:
www.cmichaelmiller.com
www.facebook.com/pages/C-Michael-Miller/123097457837462
Follow on Twitter: @CMMillerbooks
Read the Blog! www.cmichaelmiller.wordpress.com

Made in the USA
Lexington, KY
26 March 2014